Professionalism in Post-Compulsory Education and Training

T0179345

What does 'professionalism' mean for teachers and trainers in further education colleges or adult education centres? Over the last twenty years, ideas about professionalism and professional identity within the post-compulsory sector have been shaped and reshaped by successive policies, standards, and professional bodies. Yet, these ideas themselves remain controversial and continue to be the focus of debate as well as research.

This book gathers together a series of articles published over the last ten years, providing critical and research-based perspectives on professionalism within post-compulsory education and training. The twelve chapters that are presented here explore issues such as professional standards and continuing professional development and their impact on current definitions and frameworks of professionalism, as well as the policies that have shaped these processes. These are issues that are of relevance and importance not only to practitioners and researchers in the post-compulsory sector, but to anyone who is concerned with contemporary debates about what it means to be 'a professional' in education and training.

The chapters in this book were originally published as articles in *Research in Post-Compulsory Education.*

Jonathan Tummons is Associate Professor of Education at Durham University, UK. He has researched and published widely on a range of issues relating to professional, further, and higher education. His current research focuses on professional learning within medical education, and on the use of Learning Architectures theory in higher education.

Professionalism in Post-Compulsory Education and Training

Empirical and Theoretical Perspectives

Edited by
Jonathan Tummons

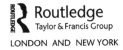
Routledge
Taylor & Francis Group

LONDON AND NEW YORK

First published 2019
by Routledge
2 Park Square, Milton Park, Abingdon, Oxon, OX14 4RN, UK

and by Routledge
52 Vanderbilt Avenue, New York, NY 10017, USA

First issued in paperback 2020

Routledge is an imprint of the Taylor & Francis Group, an informa business

© 2019 Association for Research in Post-Compulsory Education

British Library Cataloguing in Publication Data
A catalogue record for this book is available from the British Library

ISBN 13: 978-0-367-58399-6 (pbk)
ISBN 13: 978-1-138-35032-8 (hbk)

Typeset in Times New Roman
by RefineCatch Limited, Bungay, Suffolk

Publisher's Note
The publisher accepts responsibility for any inconsistencies that may have arisen during the conversion of this book from journal articles to book chapters, namely the possible inclusion of journal terminology.

Disclaimer
Every effort has been made to contact copyright holders for their permission to reprint material in this book. The publishers would be grateful to hear from any copyright holder who is not here acknowledged and will undertake to rectify any errors or omissions in future editions of this book.

Contents

Part III: Constructions of Professionalism

Citation Information

The chapters in this book were originally published in *Research in Post-Compulsory Education*. When citing this material, please use the original page numbering for each article, as follows:

Chapter 1
Performativity and professional development: the gap between policy and practice in the English further education sector
Kevin Orr
Research in Post-Compulsory Education, volume 14, issue 4 (December 2009), pp. 479–489

Chapter 2
One step forward, two steps back? The professionalisation of further education teachers in England
Norman Lucas
Research in Post-Compulsory Education, volume 18, issue 4 (December 2013), pp. 389–401

Chapter 3
Professional versus occupational models of work competence
Stan Lester
Research in Post-Compulsory Education, volume 19, issue 3 (September 2014), pp. 276–286

Chapter 4
Professionalism in vocational education: international perspectives
Liz Atkins and Jonathan Tummons
Research in Post-Compulsory Education, volume 22, issue 3 (September 2017), pp. 355–369

Chapter 5
'Square peg – round hole': the emerging professional identities of HE in FE lecturers working in a partner college network in south-west England
Rebecca Turner, Liz McKenzie and Mark Stone
Research in Post-Compulsory Education, volume 14, issue 4 (December 2009), pp. 355–368

Chapter 6

Professionalism, identity and the self: the de-moralisation of teachers in English sixth form colleges
David William Stoten
Research in Post-Compulsory Education, volume 18, issue 4 (December 2013), pp. 365–376

Chapter 7

The state of professional practice and policy in the English further education system: a view from below
Denis Gleeson, Julie Hughes, Matt O'Leary and Rob Smith
Research in Post-Compulsory Education, volume 20, issue 1 (January 2015), pp. 78–95

Chapter 8

The impact of lecturers' initial teacher training on continuing professional development needs for teaching and learning in post-compulsory education
Gary Husband
Research in Post-Compulsory Education, volume 20, issue 2 (June 2015), pp. 227–244

Chapter 9

'Nothing will prevent me from doing a good job'. The professionalisation of part-time teaching staff in further and adult education
Jill Jameson and Yvonne Hillier
Research in Post-Compulsory Education, volume 13, issue 1 (March 2008), pp. 39–53

Chapter 10

Expansive and restrictive approaches to professionalism in FE colleges: the observation of teaching and learning as a case in point
Matt O'Leary
Research in Post-Compulsory Education, volume 18, issue 4 (December 2013), pp. 348–364

Chapter 11

Professionalism: doing a good job!
Denis Feather
Research in Post-Compulsory Education, volume 19, issue 1 (January 2014), pp. 107–118

Chapter 12

Locating post-16 professionalism: public spaces as dissenting spaces
Carol Azumah Dennis
Research in Post-Compulsory Education, volume 20, issue 1 (January 2015), pp. 64–77

For any permission-related enquiries please visit:
http://www.tandfonline.com/page/help/permissions

Notes on Contributors

Liz Atkins is Professor of Vocational Education and Social Justice at Derby University, UK. Her research focuses on the school to work transitions of low-attaining youth, and how these are mediated by vocational education. She publishes widely on a range of issues related to vocational education and has also co-authored a number of practitioner texts. She is currently writing a book titled *Research Methods for Social Justice and Equity* (with Vicky Duckworth, 2018).

Carol Azumah Dennis is Senior Lecturer in Leadership and Management at the Open University, UK. Her research interests centre around three areas of specialisation: post-16 policy, professionalism and practice; leading and managing quality in vocational education; and teacher education, critical pedagogy, ethics, and social justice. Her work has been published in a wide range of journals including *Educational Management Administration & Leadership*, *International Journal of Lifelong Education*, and *Research in Post-Compulsory Education*.

Denis Feather is Senior Lecturer in the Department of Management at the University of Huddersfield, UK. His research interests lie in the study of education institutions as organisations, and how various management concepts such as 'New Performance Management' impact upon the identity of individuals, their motivation, the culture of the organisation, and values and beliefs of individuals.

Denis Gleeson is Professor Emeritus in the Centre for Education Studies at the University of Warwick, UK, and Chair of the Centre for Research and Development in Lifelong Education at the University of Wolverhampton, UK. He is a distinguished researcher, author, and teacher in further and higher education.

Yvonne Hillier is Professor of Education in the Education Research Centre at the University of Brighton, UK. She has researched issues of teaching and learning in post-compulsory education including basic skills practice, national vocational qualifications, initial teacher training, and work based learning. She is the author of *Reflective Teaching in Further, Adult and Vocational Education* (with Margaret Gregson, 2015).

Julie Hughes is Principal Lecturer and Head of the Department of Post-Compulsory Education at the University of Wolverhampton, UK. Her practice and research explores the role of Web 2.0 technologies such as e-portfolios and blogs, and their attendant dialogic pedagogies. She is particularly interested in how hybrid learning and teaching practices might support teacher transitions into FE/HE and into the workplace.

Gary Husband is Lecturer in Education at the University of Stirling, UK. His research interests are centred on the development of professional learning and leadership across all sectors of education. His ongoing work focuses on the impacts of initial training and professional learning on organisational culture and leadership development in both compulsory and post-compulsory education.

Jill Jameson is Professor of Education and Director of the Centre for Leadership and Enterprise at the University of Greenwich, UK. She is an expert in e-leadership, leadership and management in education, educational technology/e-learning, post-compulsory education/lifelong learning, and communities of practice and trust.

Stan Lester is a Consultant, Researcher and Systems Developer in professional and work-related education and development. He is the sole principal of Stan Lester Developments, and has completed or managed over 200 projects for professional bodies, universities, employers and government agencies in the UK, Europe, and beyond. He advises and supports both emerging professions, to set up systems of self-regulation; and more established ones, to review and revise standards, accreditation, and regulatory processes.

Norman Lucas is the former Head of the Lifelong Learning Academic Group at the Institute of Education, University College London, UK, where he was also Director of Post-Compulsory Teacher Education in the School of Lifelong Education and International Development. His research interests include initial teacher education and professional development, institutional management, FE incorporation and funding, and vocational education and training.

Liz McKenzie is Lecturer in Postgraduate Professional Development at the University of Plymouth, UK, where she teaches the MA in Education and the National SENCo award. Her research is centred around reflection and reflective practice; professional identities and the practice styles of HE in FE practitioners; and the experience and practice of teaching assistants.

Matt O'Leary is Professor of Education at Birmingham City University, UK. His main research interests focus on the impact of education policy on teaching and learning, professional learning, and teacher development. His books include: *Classroom observation: A guide to the effective observation of teaching and learning* (2014); *Reclaiming lesson observation: supporting excellence in teacher learning* (2016); and *Teaching Excellence in Higher Education: Challenges, Changes and the Teaching Excellence Framework* (2017).

Kevin Orr is Professor of Work and Learning and Associate Dean (Learning and Teaching) in the School of Education and Professional Development at the University of Huddersfield, UK. His research focuses on vocational education and training, teacher education and professional development in the Further Education sector, college-based higher education, and work-based learning for architects.

Rob Smith is Reader in Education at Birmingham City University, UK. His body of work explores the impact of funding and marketisation on FE provision. He has researched and written extensively in collaboration with FE and HE practitioners. He is currently developing an interdisciplinary research project looking at HE space and time focusing on the design and architecture of HEIs and their situatedness with urban settings.

Mark Stone is Head of UK Academic Partnerships at the University of Plymouth, UK, where he manages and develops existing collaborations, and builds new HE relationships in the UK.

David William Stoten is Senior Lecturer in Academic Development and Professional Support/International Distance Learning at Northumbria University, Newcastle, UK. His principal research interests are leadership, organisational theory, teaching in sixth form colleges, online learning, and self-regulated learning. Prior to entering academia, he taught in the sixth form college sector.

Jonathan Tummons is Associate Professor of Education at Durham University, UK. He has researched and published widely on a range of issues relating to professional, further, and higher education. His current research focuses on professional learning within medical education, and on the use of Learning Architectures theory in higher education.

Rebecca Turner is an Educational Developer at the University of Plymouth, UK, where she teaches on the Postgraduate Certificate in Academic Practice course and offers guidance to academic staff around all aspects of pedagogic research. Her research relates primarily to issues affecting the practice styles, identities, and research activities of lecturers working in a number of HE settings.

Introduction: what does it mean to be 'a professional'?

Jonathan Tummons

What does it mean to be 'a professional' within the post-compulsory education and training (PCET) sector? How are definitions of professionalism, as they pertain to the PCET sector, established and then sustained? Perhaps teachers and trainers within PCET see themselves as professionals and contribute in a meaningful, agentive manner to the conversations that might ensue regarding their status and qualifications, and their professional knowledge and autonomy. Or perhaps they position themselves as 'expert' in relation to different aspects of their work, relating to their occupational or subject-specialist knowledge and experience. It might be the case that some teachers have welcomed successive attempts by governments to establish new models of professionalism through introducing new qualifications, and have willingly subscribed to new professional bodies as a public indicator of the reprofessionalisation that has, it might be argued, taken place within the PCET sector. At the same time, other teachers, more or less willingly, might have disengaged from such discussions, lost in a cloud of acronyms, new compulsory training days, and changes to terms and conditions of employment.

It is almost twenty years since the first set of professional standards for teachers and trainers in PCET was published, signifying the beginning of a process (which is still underway) of professionalisation within the sector, a process that has in turn become a focus for academic research and discussion. The twelve chapters that are collected in this volume, all originally published as articles in *Research in Post-Compulsory Education*, represent research that draws on empirical as well as theoretical approaches, in order to illustrate as well as explicate the ways in which complex and troublesome issues such as professional knowledge, professionalisation, and the education of professionals, have manifested within the sector during this time. The qualitative paradigm on which these chapters all rest might be dismissed by critics as being too small in scale, too anecdotal to be sufficiently robust, but these are claims that I reject: taken together, these chapters afford a *theoretical generalisability* that provides the overarching argument presented in this volume with a sufficient warrant to be taken seriously (Alasuutari, 1995; Gobo, 2008). I shall return to a discussion of the specific themes addressed in these chapters below; for now, I wish to begin this inquiry by providing a brief, critical account of those episodes that have shaped professionalism within the PCET sector since 1999.

A brief history of (re)professionalising the further education sector

During the last two decades or so, successive government policies have been enacted that have served to define and redefine professionalism within the teaching professions at large. These processes of professionalisation have been extensively explored in relation to schools, less so in relation to further education (FE) colleges, adult and community education centres, and other providers of post-school education and training (although I deliberately exclude universities from consideration here). They can be conveniently summarised as being enrolled within a dominant discourse of education and training that is characterised by a neoliberal philosophy, enacted through successive, and ever-multiplying, policies. More specifically, they can be understood as instituting a power imbalance between teachers and the state (although the operation of the state is filtered through a series of semi-autonomous institutions), privileging compliance over critique, and characterising teaching in terms of professional competence, invariably expressed in terms of behavioural statements of occupational competency as opposed to professional knowledge. This in turn has initiated a process of professional fragmentation that has removed teachers from discussions relating to the construction or understanding of their own professionalism (Gray and Whitty, 2010). However, notwithstanding the changes to initial teacher training for schools in England that have been enacted by the Coalition and Conservative governments since 2009, the status of professional education and training for teachers in schools remains more highly developed, and more extensively researched, than the equivalent provision for teachers in further education colleges, adult education centres, community education, and work-based education settings, which here I collect together using the term 'post-compulsory education and training': PCET.

First steps in professionalisation: FEnto

It was not until the early 1990s that any serious moves toward the regulation of initial teacher training for the PCET sector were made. Several key actions were taken at this time, all of which can be seen as contributing to the ongoing process of professionalisation for the sector. In 1999, a first set of agreed professional standards was published under the auspices of the *Further Education National Training Organisation* (FEnto). National Training Organisations (NTOs) were introduced in order to define and implement relevant education and training programmes for specific sectors of trade, business, and industry. This publication followed a lengthy period of review. The standards went through eight revisions during a consultation process that involved over 200 further education colleges, 10 universities, and 23 other interested agencies (Lucas, 2004). The *Standards for Teaching and Supporting Learning in Further Education in England and Wales* (commonly referred to as 'the FEnto standards') were used in turn to inform the development of a series of new professional teaching qualifications. In 2000, the decision was taken to make these qualifications compulsory, and the publication of a statutory instrument in 2001 required these qualifications to be mapped onto the FEnto professional standards. Through aligning the teacher training curricula with the professional standards, the qualifications in question would then be benchmarked in terms of delivery, performance and assessment, all in such a way as to meet the relevant professional standard (Katz, 2000; Taylor, 1997). Between 1999 and 2002, 45 universities and five other awarding bodies (City and Guilds being the largest) had their PCET teacher education curricula endorsed by FEnto: all of these qualifications were agreed to have been constructed in such a way that upon completion (that is, successfully completing all of the required assessments) of any one of these programmes, the trainee would be deemed to have demonstrated the required threshold level of competence and knowledge necessary for a new entrant to the PCET teaching profession. 2002 also saw the establishment of the Institute for Learning (IfL), designed to be a member-led professional body, but at this time membership remained voluntary.

Criticism of the FEnto standards quickly began to emerge from both academic as well as managerial perspectives. They were criticised by university-based researchers for being overly instrumental, technicist, and undervaluing wider professional development (Elliot, 2000). They were also criticised by Ofsted, who in 2003 published their report on *The Initial Training of Further Education Teachers* (HMI 1762). According to this report, teacher education in the sector was too variable in quality and structure, and too inconsistent in design and delivery, despite the introduction of the new standards and commensurate new qualifications, to ensure consistency across the sector as a whole. A final significant criticism made by Ofsted was that PCET teacher education lacked a sufficient focus on subject-specialist pedagogy (Fisher and Webb, 2006). Nonetheless, it is perhaps uncontroversial to view the FEnto standards, in the light of any one of a number of approaches to or theories of professionalism and professionalisation, as being beneficial to the sector as a whole as well as to the teaching workforce. The requirement for teachers to be qualified and the publication of a set of standards both to codify the knowledge base of the profession and to hold that profession to account, both speak to well-established discourses of professionalism and professionalisation, processes that the sector as a whole – characterised by fragmentation, variability in teaching, and a lack of an agreed model of professional qualification and formation – badly needed at that time (Eraut, 1994; Nasta, 2007). Simply put, notwithstanding the introduction of the FEnto standards, the sector, at that time, could not comfortably be defined in terms of professionalism (Clow, 2001).

Next steps in professionalisation: LLUK and QTLS

The government paper *Equipping our teachers for the future: reforming initial teacher training for the learning and skills sector*, published one year after, and in response to, Ofsted's critical report, foreshadowed an entirely new set of professional standards and a new organisation to maintain them, an approach to defining and enacting the professional identities of teachers and trainers in the sector based on compulsory membership of the nascent Institute for Learning (IfL), and a new statutory focus on continuing as well as initial teacher education and development which would include, for the first time, mandatory subject-specialist elements. From January 2005 Lifelong Learning UK (LLUK) began operating as the body responsible for – amongst other things – the professional development of teachers and trainers in *lifelong learning*, the now-preferred nomenclature. A subsidiary organisation, Standards Verification UK (SVUK), took over the role of approving and endorsing teacher training qualifications in the post-compulsory sector that had been carried out by the now defunct FEnto. The publication of a second set of professional standards ('the LLUK standards') was followed by further statutory reform. In 2007, membership of the IfL was made compulsory for all teachers and trainers in the sector. At the same time, the IfL was also chosen (although there can not have been any serious competition) as the body that would manage both the auditing of continuing professional development (CPD) for teachers in the sector, and the process of professional formation, a sequence of post-qualification (that is, to be carried out after the completion of a Certificate in Education (CertEd) or equivalent) development activities that would lead to the award of a new professional status: Qualified Teacher, Learning and Skills (QTLS), representing the first serious attempt to establish a parity of professional esteem between teachers in schools and teachers in colleges. A teacher would receive QTLS status on completion of a compulsory teacher-training qualification, and would be required to undertake continuing professional development (CPD) in order to maintain this status, mirroring similar regulatory CPD practices across other professions.

The recommendation in the *Review of Vocational Education: the Wolf Report* of 2011 (named after Professor Alison Wolf of King's College, London, who was commissioned to write it) that holders of QTLS should be allowed to work in schools was immediately endorsed by the then Secretary of State for Education, Michael Gove, and represents the apogee of professional parity between QTLS, and Qualified Teacher Status (QTS) within schools. However, within a few months of the publication of the Wolf Report, further government legislation rendered this recommendation otiose at best. In 2012, governmental financial support for the IfL was withdrawn, the requirement for staff to register with the IfL was repealed, and professional formation leading to QTLS status was made voluntary. At the same time, routes to gaining employment in secondary schools changed. Whereas QTLS status had been positioned by the IfL as a 'passport' to the secondary sector, a point of view implicitly endorsed by the Wolf Report, the conversion of secondary schools into academies – which are not obliged to employ teaching staff with either professional qualifications or professional licenses – made the need for a QTLS 'passport' redundant. The IfL introduced a fee of £485 for the QTLS professional formation process in February 2013 as a necessary step to raise revenue, but was then closed down the following year.

The LLUK standards are generally agreed to have failed to provide a discourse of developmental, expansive professional learning for teachers and trainers in PCET, whose training continued to be seen as a 'second thought' by policy makers (Lucas and Nasta, 2010). The push to introduce subject-specialist pedagogy within the PCET teacher-training curriculum was effectively restricted to the provision of subject-specialist mentoring, characterised by inconsistency of implementation between different providers, and conflicting discourses of professionalism. Mentoring was intended as the process through which subject-specialist pedagogic development might be embedded within a generic teacher-training qualification (Fisher and Webb, 2006). However, concerns were quickly raised that the provision of mentoring in further education should not be unproblematically assumed to be as straightforward to implement and evaluate as schools-based mentoring for newly qualified school teachers, not least due to the considerable organisational complexity of the FE sector (Hankey, 2004). Further concerns related to the extent to which mentoring might be implemented according to a judgemental as opposed to developmental model, due to the need to audit and evaluate the process (Ingleby and Tummons, 2012; Tedder and Lawy, 2009). Nor did the IfL succeed in establishing itself as a serious advocate for practitioners within the sector, and it received criticism for maintaining a leadership group that was too remote from the membership. At the same time, there were disagreements with the University and College Union (UCU) over fees and with the Association of Colleges (AoC) regarding disciplinary measures against staff for non-payment of IfL membership fees during the period of compulsory membership.

Further steps in professionalisation: ETF

After the demise of the IfL in 2014, the key tasks of managing the QTLS professional formation process and stewarding a new set of professional standards for teachers in PCET fell to the Education and Training Foundation (ETF) and a subsidiary organisation for members, the Society for Education and Training (SET). The *Professional Standards for Teachers and Trainers in Education and Training* framework is significantly shorter than the two previous sets of standards: indeed, the new ETF framework is shorter in total than any one of the six domains of practice that made up the LLUK standards. The ETF has been criticised for a narrowing of focus since its inception. In March 2018, the Association of Employment and Learning Providers, a member-led body that is concerned primarily with the provision of apprenticeships, withdrew from its governance role within the ETF, arguing that the ETF had become too focussed on the mainstream FE sector at the expense of the wider PCET sector, and that the relationship between the ETF and the Department for Education (DfE), as the main funding provider, threatened the notion of the body being run by the sector and for the sector. At the same time, the ETF has continued a programme of funding professional development and networking events for managers and governors as well as teachers and trainers, opportunities for small-scale funded research through a partnership with the University of Sunderland (a long-standing HE provider of initial teacher-training for the sector), and from 2015 to 2017 was a key stakeholder in the Area Review of FE Colleges. The QTLS process, now once again voluntary, was supplemented in 2017 by a new professional formation process, *Advanced Teacher Status* (ATS) which, on completion, will also confer Chartered Teacher Status from the Chartered College of Teaching.

So what is the current condition of professionalism within the FE sector? We find that professional qualifications are now – once again – voluntary, not compulsory: a voluntarism that has been justified in terms of employer-led flexibility and individual choice, characteristic of the neoliberal discourse within which the sector finds itself. We find a sector that is now working with the third set of professional standards to have been imposed on the teaching workforce over the last twenty years. Teacher education for the sector remains variable in terms of academic levels, credit structures, and assessment regimes (Lucas, Nasta and Rogers, 2012). It remains underfunded, and poorly integrated within wider human resources structures within the college sector, a reflection of the fragmented nature of the FE landscape (O'Dwyer and Thorpe, 2013). Entry to the profession (if it is, indeed, a 'profession') continues to be characterised as much by the ad-hoc practices of the 'long interview' (Gleeson and James, 2007), of part-time and/or precarious employment and in-service qualifications, rather than full-time pre-service qualifications and a formalised process of professional probation. One professional body has come and gone, and another – distinctly employer-led rather than member-led – has taken its place (Tummons, 2014a). Professional qualifications continue to be characterised by a lack of propositional knowledge (Loo, 2014), and to rest on a teacher-training curriculum that remains relatively unchanged (Tummons, 2014b). Teachers within the sector remain ambiguous in their awareness of and responses to, professional standards as public documents that purport to shape their profession (Tummons, 2016). The work done by FE teachers continues to intensify, as it has done during the last twenty years, to include tutorial, pastoral and wider support roles (Avis and Bathmaker, 2004; Robson and Bailey, 2009). Policy makers continue simultaneously to marginalise the sector through the withdrawal of financial and political capital, and discombobulate the sector through constant changes in funding mechanisms and regulatory systems (Bailey and Unwin, 2014; Finlay et al., 2007; Robson, 1998).

From a 'top-down' perspective, the current uncertain condition of professionalism and professionalisation within PCET can be seen as being symptomatic of a sector that is, more widely, as fragmented and vulnerable to political and economic change as it has ever been. This is not, however, to deny the serious intent that lies behind the choices made by teachers in colleges or adult education centres to achieve QTLS status, or to study for a higher degree, or to engage in practitioner research. Rather, it is to acknowledge the limitations placed on autonomous models of professionalism by the political and financial structures that shape the sector at large.

Researching professionalism and professionalisation

Notwithstanding the fact that the PCET sector is relatively under-researched in comparison to schools and universities, there has been a steady increase in robust empirical as well as conceptual research relating to the sector more generally, and the specific problems of professionalism and professionalisation more specifically, in recent years. Within this field, the journal *Research in Post-Compulsory Education* (*RPCE*) has, for over twenty years, made a significant contribution, publishing work from emerging as well as established researchers, from increasingly diverse perspectives.

Part one of this collection is titled *Professionalism: standards and policies*, and consists of four chapters that, taken together, provide an account of the development of teaching standards within the sector during the last twenty years, whilst also drawing on longer-established debates on the nature of professional work and knowledge. In the second part, *Professional Identities*, the focus shifts from policy to practitioners: the four chapters in this section explore complex notions of professional identity within and across a range of institutional fields or contexts. And in part three, *Constructions of Professionalism*, contrasting, and sometimes conflicting, models and discourses of professionalism are evaluated and theorised. Taken together – and it is important not to balkanise these three themes but to acknowledge that many themes cut across the collection as a whole – these twelve chapters report on research that reflects the diversity of not only the PCET sector but also the kinds of research work being currently undertaken: further education lecturers, adult education tutors, sixth form lecturers and higher education in further education staff (HE in FE) are all represented here, as are a range of approaches to research, including empirical, policy, and theoretical/conceptual research. The four chapters that make up each part of this collection are presented chronologically, in order to highlight the persistence of many of the questions and debates that are to be found within them. Many of these questions are discussed by several of the authors represented here, although not always from the same point of view or drawing on the same kinds of research. These chapters do not represent a consensus in terms of research findings or policy recommendations, but they do represent a robust and coherent field of research. And it is to a holistic discussion of the chapters that constitute each of the three parts of this collection that I now turn.

Professionalism: standards and policies

The starting point for our inquiry is made up of three related elements: firstly, the role of policy (including not only government policy, but also policy at organisational and/or institutional levels) in the reification of professional standards; secondly, the imposition of performativity cultures within the workplace; and thirdly, conflicting discourses of professionalism. Taken together, the four chapters that are presented here provide an account that explicates top-down, managerialist, dominant discourses of professionalism that can be seen to have an impact on the everyday work of teachers and trainers, and that are to be contrasted with developmental or emancipatory models of professionalism.

The first chapter, by Kevin Orr, consists of an account of the continuing professional development (CPD) framework of the IfL. Combining an analysis of the CPD framework with the results of a small-scale empirical inquiry, Orr positions the CPD requirements of the IfL as a conduit to a more wide-reaching exploration of performativity cultures within the FE sector (where his research is located) whilst simultaneously exposing the sclerotic nature of the policy that surrounded the CPD framework. Within this performativity culture, any potential for CPD to provide meaningful professional development and enhancement of professional knowledge and/or practice is either sidelined by policies where individual CPD is neglected in favour of staff development that follows organisational priorities, or neglected by practitioners who lack meaningful institutional support for their own further professional learning and development. Within this discourse of performativity, CPD becomes reduced to activities that can be straightforwardly audited.

The impact of an ever-changing policy landscape upon teachers in FE is further explored in the chapter by Norman Lucas. In discussing the dismantling of LLUK and the IfL, and predicting (accurately) a return to voluntarism for teacher education within the sector, Lucas focuses on Ofsted's critique of the paucity of subject-specialist pedagogy (in HMI 1762, as previously discussed) and the subsequent development of mentoring for trainee teachers in colleges (like the preceding chapter, Lucas' paper is also situated within FE). Drawing on his own prior empirical research, Lucas demonstrates the gap between rhetoric and reality for teacher development within the LLUK/ QTLS framework, which he characterises as uneven and lacking sufficient institutional support from not only the colleges where trainees worked, but also the awarding bodies that provided the teaching qualifications. Noting the lack of policy or institutional interest in the informal workplace learning of new FE teachers and trainers, Lucas concludes that the FEnto and LLUK regimes failed either to improve teaching standards or to enhance teacher professionalism within the sector.

The third chapter, by Stan Lester, moves our inquiry away from the further education sector and towards a broader field of work competence, locating professional competence and occupational competence as distinct constructs with distinct bodies of professional capability and capacity. Lester's synthesis of professional frameworks from a range of different contexts serves to generate a series of stark contrasts between these wider discourses of professionalism, and the model of professionalism evidenced within the FE sector as already outlined by both Orr and Lucas. The model of professionalism that Lester explicates – a model resting on not only professional standards but also on professional ethics (the latter, as also noted by Lucas, having been studiously avoided by the IfL), on wider professional capability, and on entry to a profession rather than to a specific job role – emerges in stark contrast to the model presented by Orr in particular as distorted by the requirements of audit and by both Orr and Lucas as in thrall to the vicissitudes of policy.

Liz Atkins and I co-wrote the fourth chapter in this section, in which we set out to bring the conversation surrounding professional standards up-to-date through exploring the ETF framework and juxtaposing this with equivalent standards in Australia. We explored both qualifications as well as professional frameworks in Australia (the latter, it is important to note, are at state and not national level). We concluded that in both the UK and Australia there was a lack of any serious discussion of a propositional knowledge base for teachers in FE/VET (vocational education and training – the term used in Australia) within the competency-based models of professionalism that prevail in both contexts. The ETF framework discusses professional knowledge, professional development, professional behaviour, professional learning, and professional conduct – but provides no definitions for these contested terms; nor are they pinned to a professional ethos or philosophy, in stark contrast to the more mature models of professionalism explored by Lester.

In this first part of our inquiry, therefore, we find a further education sector that exhibits at best a restricted, if not diminished, model of professionalism, a model that has emerged over time and through an at times bewildering succession of regulatory frameworks, painstakingly mapped onto successive – and increasingly brief – sets of professional standards that remain at an occupational, competence-based level, that eschew any serious discussion of the developmental nature of professional knowledge and expertise, and that foreground bureaucratic compliance at the expense of individual agency. With the PCET sector in such a state of fragmentation, as clearly demonstrated by Lucas, it is perhaps unsurprising that successive iterations of professional standards have been relatively ineffectual in engendering an autonomous professionalism resting on expertise and capability.

Professional identities

The second stage of our inquiry shifts our focus towards the lived experience of teachers and trainers in different parts of the PCET sector: FE provision, Higher Education in Further Education (HE in FE) provision, and sixth form colleges. These contexts are all quite distinct, but nonetheless merit consideration alongside each other, exhibiting as they do a number of shared characteristics that can be brought together within an analysis of the impact on enacted professional identities of contemporary cultures of audit and accountability. The four chapters that are presented here combine theoretical as well as empirical perspectives, identifying the dominant managerialist discourses that impact on teachers' working lives, but also identifying the ways in which these same teachers recognise these discourses and go on to reject them as antithetical to their own constructions of professionalism.

The first chapter is by Rebecca Turner, Liz McKenzie, and Mark Stone, and rests on an interview-based study of HE in FE lecturers. Through exploring lecturers' responses to the distinct demands of the two professional contexts within which they work, comparing their roles in 'mainstream' FE with their roles in college-based university provision, Turner and her colleagues highlight the differences between the two teaching cultures. For the lecturers represented here, teaching within the HE curriculum is characterised by higher levels of professional autonomy, greater opportunities for recognition as subject-specialists, and a commitment to a widening participation ethos (reflecting broader discourses within the HE in FE sector as a whole (Tummons et al., 2013)), characterised here as a model of *hybrid professionalism* that falls, sometimes uncomfortably, between the work of the university lecturer as focussed on research and subject expertise (a view that is, arguably, somewhat idealised) and the work of the college lecturer as having to balance the requirements of the university partner with the more managerial requirements of the college.

The research participants in David Stoten's survey-based study of teachers in three different sixth form colleges are likewise cognisant of the audit cultures that impact on their own constructions of professionalism. Drawing on the work of Jürgen Habermas, and specifically on the notion of the diminished personal autonomy of the self, which is conceptualised as a response to the audit culture professionalism that is one of the consequences of New Public Management (NPM) within education, Stoten demonstrates that teachers recognise the changing ideological contexts of their work. Some exhibit agency through constructing their own ethical frameworks in opposition to the business model of education that they encounter in practice, whilst others exhibit varying degrees of professional alienation, describing themselves as being disempowered by the prevailing cultures of the neoliberal workplace.

The neoliberal workplace also serves as a locus for inquiry within the chapter by Denis Gleeson, Julie Hughes, Matt O'Leary, and Rob Smith. Once again drawing on prior conceptual as well as empirical research, Gleeson et al. posit two distinct identities for teachers in further education colleges, contrasting the empowered professional with the education worker. The former is characterised by a strong commitment to a dual professionalism (Orr and Simmons, 2010) that foregrounds vocational pedagogy in opposition to the latter, working within a technicist model of professionalism that is encouraged by an uncritical adherence to inspection criteria and other quality assurance processes on the part of college managers and leaders. Within this fragmented workplace, Gleeson and colleagues argue that the many positive outcomes for learners in FE derive to a significant degree from the expertise of FE teachers and their willingness to expand their responsibilities and take on pastoral roles – aspects of professionalism that are absent from the quality assurance discourses that measure teachers' work through lesson observations.

The final chapter in this section, by Gary Husband, also foregrounds expertise and experience in the construction of a strong professional identity, critically appraising the roles of initial teacher training and continuing professional development on the individual. Drawing on an interview-based study carried out across two FE colleges, Husband demonstrates the need for ongoing professional learning after a period of initial training, in order to allow teachers to develop expertise and skill in those aspects of teaching in FE that, from the perspectives of the practitioners who were interviewed, were only inadequately covered during teacher training. Mirroring the wider literature on professional learning, Husband positions initial teacher education as a necessary element of professional formation, but at a threshold level that obligates the practitioner to continue their professional learning once in the workplace.

In this second part of our inquiry, therefore, we find teachers and trainers from across a range of PCET contexts – 'mainstream' FE, HE in FE, and sixth form colleges – making sense of their own, emergent, notions of professionalism in contrast to the dominant discourses of audit culture professionalism that is found across the sector. This audit culture professionalism restricts the practitioner in several ways: through generating a fractured and casualised workforce and through diminishing personal autonomy, reducing the practitioner to an education worker. At the same time, we also find practitioners exercising agency in order to resist this managerialist discourse: through promulgating their own ethical frameworks, enhancing their own professional identities through developing expertise, and where possible resisting managerial approaches to professional development and training. Simply put, these four chapters provide evidence of traces of resistance to the New Public Management that has driven the (re)professionalisation of PCET in recent times.

Constructions of professionalism

The third and final stage of our inquiry picks up on the theme of resistance to the dominant managerial discourse and seeks to locate these moments of resistance within emergent models of autonomic professionalism as enacted and voiced by the social actors involved: the teachers and trainers. Taken together, the four chapters that make up this final strand of our discussion continue to offer a pluralist view of PCET, representing, through the reporting of empirical research, the voices of practitioners in not only 'mainstream' FE but also HE in FE and, introducing a new element to our depiction of the sector, tutors working in adult and community learning. These chapters move our analysis beyond the ways in which practitioners resist audit professionalism and towards ways of defining an autonomous professionalism.

The first chapter in this section is by Jill Jameson and Yvonne Hillier, and draws on a survey of hourly-paid tutors in adult and community education (ACE) to explore the ways in which their 'part-timeness' affords patterns of flexibility and responsibility at work that in turn contribute to an autonomous construction of professionalism. Drawing broadly on a sociocultural epistemology and ontology, Jameson and Hillier contrast the agency of part-time tutors with the managerial restrictions of full-time teachers. For the tutors in ACE, professionalism resides in their obligation to their students and in the autonomy that derives from their peripheral positions within the organisations for which they teach. This is a professionalism that derives from prac-tice, not from adherence to an organisation or from contractual status.

Matt O'Leary's chapter draws on a large mixed methods study of lesson observa-tions in the FE sector. Focussing on just two colleges derived from the original research sample of ten colleges and 500 members of staff, O'Leary provides accounts from staff at all levels – managers, teachers, observers, and mentors – of two contrasting organisational approaches to the observation process. At the first site, observation is collaborative, negotiated and transparent, embedded within a broader and more mean-ingful process of professional development, driven by the individual needs of the member of staff being observed. The autonomy and agency of the teacher are preserved within a culture that positions observation as a developmental tool, not a judgemental one. At the second site, by contrast, the observation of teaching and learning process is combative rather than supportive, imposed and not welcomed, characterised by a lack of trust on the part of managers towards those doing the observations, supporting a mentoring culture that is punitive, forced on teachers who are constructed as 'failing' by the observation process.

In the third chapter of this section of our inquiry, our focus shifts once again to the sometimes professionally ambiguous culture of HE in FE. Echoing the sense of HE in FE being separate from mainstream FE explicated in the earlier chapter by Rebecca Turner and colleagues, Denis Feather's interview-based study foregrounds a number of related themes that HE in FE staff position as being important elements of their personal codes of professional behaviour. In contrast to the target cultures and busi-ness models of education that colleges are obligated to adopt by successive govern-ment policies and initiatives, HE in FE staff argue that autonomy, expertise through qualifications, being trusted, and staying up-to-date are what it means to be profes-sional, although a more universal definition of 'professionalism' remains elusive and difficult to define.

The chapter by Carol Azumah Dennis that completes this section likewise focuses on the ways in which teachers themselves discuss what does, and what does not, constitute being a professional. Constructing empirical data through analysing an online forum managed by the *Times Educational Supplement*, Dennis conceptualises this online space as a locus for the discursive explication of professionalism by teachers, focussing specifically on online discussions by teachers in both the UK and the USA (although it is the responses of the former that are of particular salience to the present inquiry) relating to post-qualification professional registration. Dennis argues that for the teachers in her study, membership – whether mandatory or not – of a professional asso-ciation did not generate a sense of professionalism or an ethos of professional conduct, not least when the association in question came into being due to legislation rather than due to a member-led process of organisation.

In this third part of our inquiry, therefore, we find a consensus emerging from across institutional boundaries (FE, HE in FE, ACE) and from practitioners holding different occupational statuses (full-time teachers, part-time hourly paid teachers, managers). Of equal importance is the temporal dimension afforded by these chapters: Jameson and Hillier report on empirical research that was originally conducted over a decade ago, and yet the themes that they address are still relevant to more recent research. What is noteworthy here is the consistency of the discourse offered by practitioners, who construct their professional identities, their personal codes of what it means to be 'a professional' not in terms of membership of an association or uncritical adherence to organisational or governmental target cultures, but in terms of being trusted to do their work, of being given autonomy, of a professionalism rooted in expertise and qualifications and an ethic of care to their students and apprentices.

Conclusion: what does it mean to be 'a professional'

Teachers, trainers and tutors within the PCET sector – here taken to include lecturers in further education colleges, in adult and community education, in sixth form colleges, and in HE in FE – share much common ground in constructing their own working identities in terms of a professional ethos, notwithstanding the difficulties that are to be found in attempting to produce a single and fixed definition of 'professionalism'. Invariably rejecting the business model of education that is characteristic of the contemporary neoliberal discourse of public policy more widely, and of educational provision more specifically, teachers and trainers place their expertise and specialist qualifications alongside their willingness to embrace the wider supportive and pastoral work, the *emotional labour*, that their ethic of care compels them to attend to. This is a form of supererogatory professionalism, therefore, where many teachers and trainers are willing to extend their work beyond their subject specialism. At the same time, they attend to the bureaucratic, managerial demands of their workplaces, sometimes more-or-less willingly, invariably strategically, whilst simultaneously ring-fencing their pedagogic practice as a locus for autonomy. Organisational policies, professional bodies and codes of practice or standards are not ignored; nor are they enthusiastically embraced. It is in teachers' work with their students and their deserved pride in their knowledge and expertise, not in the imposed structures of governments, managers and imposed employer-led organisations, that the traces of an emancipatory professionalism are to be found.

References

Alasuutari, P. 1995. *Researching Culture: qualitative method and cultural studies.* London: Sage.
Avis, J. and A. M. Bathmaker. 2004. The politics of care: emotional labour and trainee further education lecturers. *Journal of Vocational Education and Training* 56(1): 5–20.
Bailey, B. and L. Unwin. 2014. Continuity and change in English further education: a century of voluntarism and permissive adaptability. *British Journal of Educational Studies* 62(4): 449–464.
Clow, R. 2001. Further education teachers' constructions of professionalism. *Journal of Vocational Education and Training* 53(3): 407–420.
Elliott, G. 2000. Accrediting lecturers using competence-based approaches: a cautionary tale. In Gray, D. and C. Griffin, (eds.) *Post-compulsory Education and the New Millennium*. London: Jessica Kingsley.
Eraut, M. 1994. *Developing Professional Knowledge and Competence*. Abingdon: Routledge-Falmer.

Finlay, I., K. Spours, R. Steer, F. Coffield, M. Gregson, and A. Hodgson. 2007. 'The Heart of What We Do': policies on teaching, learning and assessment in the learning and skills sector. *Journal of Vocational Education and Training* 59(2): 137–153.

Fisher, R. and K. Webb. 2006. Subject specialist pedagogy and initial teacher training for the learning and skills sector in England: the context, a response and some critical issues. *Journal of Further and Higher Education* 30(4): 337–349.

Gleeson, D. and D. James. 2007. The paradox of professionalism in English further education: a TLC project perspective. *Educational Review* 59(4): 451–467.

Gobo, G. 2008. Reconceptualising generalisation: old issues in a new frame. In Alasuutari, A., L. Bickman, and J. Brannen, (eds.) *The Sage Handbook of Social Research Methods*. London: Sage.

Gray, S. and G. Whitty. 2010. Social trajectories or disrupted identities? Changing and competing models of teacher professionalism under New Labour. *Cambridge Journal of Education* 40(1): 5–23.

Hankey, J. 2004. The good, the bad and other considerations: reflections on mentoring trainee teachers in post-compulsory education. *Research in Post-Compulsory Education* 9(3): 389–400.

Ingleby, E. and J. Tummons. 2012. Repositioning professionalism: teachers, mentors, policy and praxis. *Research in Post-Compulsory Education* 17(2): 163–178.

Katz, T. 2000. University education for developing professional practice. In Bourner, T., T. Katz, and D. Watson, (eds.) *New Directions in Professional Higher Education*, 19–32. Buckingham: Open University Press/Society for Research into Higher Education.

Loo, S. 2014. Placing 'knowledge' in teacher education in the English further education sector: an alternative approach based on collaboration and evidence-based research. *British Journal of Educational Studies* 62(3): 337–354.

Lucas, N. 2004. The 'FENTO Fandango': national standards, compulsory teaching qualifications and the growing regulation of FE teachers. *Journal of Further and Higher Education* 28(1): 35–51.

Lucas, N. and T. Nasta. 2010. State regulation and the professionalisation of further education teachers: a comparison with schools and HE. *Journal of Vocational Education and Training* 62(4): 441–454.

Lucas, N., T. Nasta, and L. Rogers. 2012. From fragmentation to chaos? The regulation of initial teacher education in further education. *British Educational Research Journal* 38(4): 677–695.

Nasta, T. 2007. Translating national standards into practice for the initial training of further education (FE) teachers in England. *Research in Post-Compulsory Education* 12(1): 1–17.

O'Dwyer, A. and A. Thorpe. 2013. Managers' understandings of supporting teachers with specific learning disabilities: macro and micro understanding in the English Further Education sector. *Cambridge Journal of Education* 43(1): 89–105.

Orr, K. and R. Simmons. 2010. Dual identities: the in-service teacher trainee experience in the English further education sector. *Journal of Vocational Education and Training* 62(1): 75–88.

Robson, J. 1998. A profession in crisis: status, culture and identity in the further education college. *Journal of Vocational Education and Training* 50(4): 585–607.

Robson, J. and B. Bailey. 2009. 'Bowing from the heart': an investigation into discourses of professionalism and the work of caring for students in further education. *British Educational Research Journal* 35(1): 99–117.

Taylor, I. 1997. *Developing Learning in Professional Education.* Buckingham: Open University Press/Society for Research into Higher Education.

Tedder, M. and R. Lawy. 2009. The pursuit of 'excellence': mentoring in further education initial teacher training in England. *Journal of Vocational Education and Training* 61(4): 413–429.

Tummons, J. 2014a. The textual representation of professionalism: problematising professional standards for teachers in the UK lifelong learning sector. *Research in Post-Compulsory Education* 19(1): 33–44.

Tummons, J. 2014b. Professional standards in teacher education: tracing discourses of professionalism through the analysis of textbooks. *Research in Post-Compulsory Education* 19(4): 417–432.

Tummons, J. 2016. 'Very positive' or 'vague and detached'? Unpacking ambiguities in further education teachers' responses to professional standards in England. *Research in Post-Compulsory Education* 21(4): 346–359.

Tummons, J., K. Orr, and L. Atkins. 2013. *Teaching higher education courses in further education colleges.* London: SAGE/Learning Matters.

Performativity and professional development: the gap between policy and practice in the English further education sector

Kevin Orr

The New Labour government identified the further education (FE) sector as a vehicle to deliver its central policies on social justice and economic competitiveness in England, which has led to a torrent of initiatives that have increased central scrutiny and control over FE. Although the connections between social justice, economic competitiveness and education are hegemonic in mainstream British politics, they are unfounded. Therefore, FE can only fail to deliver fully the government's central programme. Thus, a gap exists between policy initiatives and practice in colleges even, paradoxically, where reforms are ostensibly successful. In order to illustrate this gap and how it is maintained this paper considers one specific reform: the statutory obligation for teachers in English FE colleges to undertake 30 hours of continuing professional development (CPD) annually. Evidence from small-scale exploratory research suggests that this initiative has had little impact on patterns of CPD, though the government's quantifiable targets are being systematically met. This paper argues that a symbiosis of performativity has evolved where the government produces targets and colleges produce mechanisms to 'evidence' their achievement, separate to any change in practice and thus maintaining the gap between policy and practice.

Introduction

'Whatever else you could say about Labour's educational policies there is certainly no shortage of them' (Ball 2008, 86).

Over three million learners (Foster 2005, vi) attend English further education (FE) colleges which are part of a heterogeneous sector that has been described as what is not school and not university (Kennedy 1997, 1), though even those boundaries are becoming less defined. It remains the sector where the majority of vocational training and adult education takes place, as well as academic study between the ages of 16 and 18. The New Labour government, elected in 1997, identified FE as a means to deliver two central policies in England: social justice through widening participation in education; and enhancing national economic competitiveness through improving the workforce's skills (Orr 2008). Therefore, while previous governments largely neglected FE (Lucas 2004, 35), New Labour has increasingly scrutinised and controlled colleges and staff; a process which is apparent in the government's *Workforce Strategy for the*

Further Education System in England, 2007–2012 (Lifelong Learning UK [LLUK] 2008a). This strategy includes the introduction of a statutory annual period of continuing professional development (CPD) for teachers in FE colleges, on which this paper focuses. From September 2007 each teacher must carry out and record 30 hours of CPD each year in order to maintain their licence to practise (Institute for Learning [IfL] 2009, 14).

Finlay et al. (2007, 138) describe *policy* as a 'loose term' which includes: 'value commitments, strategic objectives and operational instruments and structures at national, regional, local and institutional levels'.

Such a catholic understanding of policy is necessary within FE where there is a plethora of national and local agencies, bodies and institutions. As part of their wide-ranging and detailed research into the impact of policy in the learning and skills sector in England, Coffield et al. (2008, 15–17) created an organigram of the sector which they describe as looking 'more like the chart of the internal wiring of an advanced computer than the outline of a "streamlined", coherent sector'. This complexity has arisen partly because of the diversity of the sector and its conflicting constituencies (Coffield et al. 2007, 735), but also because policy has been laid on policy, and for New Labour that has meant organisation laid upon organisation. So, CPD in FE over the past decade has been under the direction of five different government departments and at least five different government-funded agencies. Besides these is the nominally independent professional body for teaching staff in FE, the IfL, whose website (IfL 2008) helpfully contains 250 acronyms used in the sector. Note, though, that IfL 'do not expect [this list] to be comprehensive'. Such complexity itself becomes an important factor in the implementation of any policy initiative.

Using definitions developed by Steer et al. (2007, 177) policy drivers are the broadly described aims while a policy lever, is 'shorthand for the wide array of functional mechanisms through which government and its agencies seek to implement policies'. The use of targets for FE colleges is one such policy lever. In order to demonstrate how policy levers become detached from the changes they are meant to force, I consider the targets related to the CPD reform. This reform demonstrates three aspects of the government's approach to FE. Firstly, efforts to direct the sector closely have had the effect of reducing professional autonomy and trust by increasing centralised accountability. Secondly, the means to measure the initiative's success have diverged from the intended change in colleges as systems to record the achievement of targets are introduced and prioritised. Finally, despite its ostensible success through achievement of targets, the initiative has changed little in practice.

This paper draws on small-scale qualitative research into the introduction of compulsory CPD to demonstrate how a symbiosis of performativity has evolved from government reforms, which indicates how the gap between national initiatives and local practice is perpetuated. Questionnaires were submitted to 42 human resources managers, teacher-trainers and others who identified themselves as having responsibility for staff development and CPD at FE organisations in the north of England in October 2008. This was just over a year after the introduction of the CPD initiative. Twenty-nine completed questionnaires were returned from staff at 21 organisations. These questionnaires sought their attitudes towards compulsory CPD and descriptions of how their organisations were implementing the reform. Participants were specifically asked to describe how their organisation was demonstrating achievement of the government's targets relating to CPD. This research provides a snapshot picture of the early trajectory of the CPD reform, which suggests how national policy can be distorted by local implementation and by the need to demonstrate achievement of targets. Before discussing the findings from these local FE organisations in more detail, I consider the development of national policy for FE which has shaped how those organisations responded to the CPD reform.

FE policy under New Labour

Tomlinson (2001, 112) stressed the 'continuities and similarities' between the approaches to post-16 education of the Conservative and New Labour governments, but the new government recognised the need for reform in the 1999 White Paper, *Learning to Succeed: A New Framework for Post-16 Learning*:

> There is too much duplication, confusion and bureaucracy in the current system. Too little money actually reaches learners and employers, too much is tied up in bureaucracy. There is an absence of effective co-ordination or strategic planning. The system has insufficient focus on skill and employer needs at national, regional and local levels. (Department for Education and Employment [DfEE] 1999, 21)

Apparently, FE was broken and needed fixing before it could carry New Labour's policies, which led to the current government spending more time and effort on the sector than any previous one. In 2004 Lucas (2004, 35) wrote:

> It is probably true that in the last five years or so there has been more regulation and government policy concerned with raising the standards of teaching in further education than ever before.

The same statement could be made about the five years that followed for reasons that lie at the heart of the New Labour project. Hall (2003, 6) accused New Labour of speaking 'with forked tongue' by rhetorically combining economic neo-liberalism with their more social-democratic strand. However, for New Labour the connections between education and training, economic growth and social justice are simply unquestionable. These connections, considered more fully later, are rhetorically positioned to be unassailable and so broach no argument nor require any evidence because there is, apparently, no alternative. Smith (1994, 37; cited in Avis 2003, 317) describes the process of hegemony, which can be related to educational policy in this area:

> A hegemonic project does not dominate political subjects: it does not reduce political subjects to pure obedience and it does not even require their unequivocal support for its specific demands. It pursues, instead, a far more subtle goal, namely the vision of the social order as the social order itself.

> To describe a political project as hegemonic, then, is not to say that a majority of the electorate explicitly supports its policies, but to say that there appears to be no other alternative to this project's vision of society.

The orthodoxy that makes education an aspect of economic policy is part of what Ball (1999, 204, original emphasis) has called a 'powerful, coherent *policyscape*', where social justice is aligned with economic competitiveness, as apparent in New Labour's statements. David Blunkett, the first New Labour Secretary of State for Education, wrote in the foreword to the government Green Paper in 1998:

> Learning is the key to prosperity – for each of us as individuals, as well as for the nation as a whole. Investment in human capital will be the foundation of success in the knowledge-based global economy of the twenty-first century. This is why the Government has put learning at the heart of its ambition. (DfEE 1998, 1)

Seven years later in 2005 Bill Rammell, then British minister of state for Higher Education and Lifelong Learning claimed: 'Further Education is the engine room for skills and social justice in this country' (Learning and Skills Council 2005, 1), and he was among ministers who welcomed the Leitch Review of Skills published in 2006 which asserted: 'where skills were once **a** key driver of prosperity and fairness, they are now **the** key driver' (Leitch 2006, 46, original emphases). That same year Prime Minister Tony Blair wrote in the foreword to a Government White Paper:

> Our economic future depends on our productivity as a nation. That requires a labour force with skills to match the best in the world…
>
> The colleges and training providers that make up the Further Education sector are central to achieving that ambition… But at present, Further Education is not achieving its full potential as the powerhouse of a high skills economy. (Department for Education and Skills [DfES] 2006)

This extract indicates the continued importance to the government of the economic role of FE, though exactly what 'high skills' are is not specified, and it indicates that ministers still considered FE not to be working properly. The perceived failure of FE to achieve 'its full potential' led to increasing the centralised accountability of FE teachers, which Morris (2001, 26) celebrated in relation to school teachers in a speech made while she was Minister of Education:

> We do now have an accountable profession. Performance tables, the inspection system, performance management, examination and assessment arrangements, procedures for tackling school weaknesses, all contribute to the effective accountability of teachers and headteachers.

The Workforce Strategy for the Further Education System in England, 2007–2012, which includes mandatory annual CPD, can be understood within this context of perceived failure leading to increased accountability. One important element of this strategy is the *New Overarching Professional Standards for Teachers, Tutors and Trainers in the Lifelong Learning Sector,* which contain 190 statements of the 'skills, knowledge and attributes' (LLUK 2006, ii) required by those who work in the sector, including a commitment to: '[u]sing a range of learning resources to support learners' (LLUK 2006, 4); and the requirement to '[s]tructure and present information clearly and effectively' (LLUK 2006, 5). The length of these standards and their banal specification of practice contrast unfavourably with the equivalent documents covering the schools and HE sectors which briefly set out broad professional values and do not attempt to prescribe classroom activities (Orr 2008, 103). The content and tenor of the documents that relate to FE suggest what Avis (2003, 315) termed 'a truncated model of trust', but why do policymakers treat FE in such a manner? Certainly this most heterogeneous sector is important to the government, as I have argued, yet Coffield et al. (2008, 4) argue that those with authority fail to understand the sector because, 'with a few exceptions, neither they nor their children have ever passed through it'. For the same reason the FE sector does not have the lobbying strength of schools and universities and so is more susceptible to the activities of new ministers wishing to make their own mark. Nonetheless, while legislation has rained down upon FE there is a gap between what may be planned by government reform and what it achieves in practice as one initiative demands another to achieve what the former failed to. This pattern results from the government's ideological investment in the links between education and training, social justice and economic competitiveness.

Despite its hegemony in mainstream British politics, this conjoining of educational, economic and social policy has been subject to excoriating criticism from, among others, Coffield (1999), Rikowski (2001) and Avis (2007), who have found that the orthodoxy has no foundation in evidence. Reporting on a recent major research project into education, globalisation and the knowledge economy, Brown, Lauder and Ashton (2008, 17) found that 'while the skills of the workforce remain important, they are not a source of decisive competitive advantage'. Moreover, they found that the expansion of access to Higher Education (HE) in the UK 'has failed to narrow income inequalities even amongst university graduates'. Therefore, the government is subjecting FE to ever-greater scrutiny and accountability for what cannot be accomplished through education and training alone. There is a fundamental discrepancy between the government's intention for FE and what FE can achieve, no matter how efficient the sector is. The White Paper in which Blair wrote the foreword quoted previously was also the document that first introduced compulsory CPD for all staff in FE; another means to fix a broken FE sector.

CPD and workforce strategy

The shift from voluntary to compulsory CPD in FE is only the most prominent aspect of *The Workforce Strategy* which:

> …is intended to help shape the further education workforce of the future in England. By providing a national framework, it is intended to support all colleges and learning providers to implement their own local workforce plans to support the delivery of excellent provision for young people, adults and employers. (LLUK 2008a, 6)

The government minister Bill Rammell (LLUK 2008a, 4) praised the progress of staff in FE in his foreword to the initiative before warning that given current and future developments: 'All those who lead and work in the sector will need to move up a gear'. David Hunter, chief executive of LLUK (LLUK 2008a, 5) wrote in his foreword: 'There is already much success to celebrate and the Further Education Sector workforce can be rightly proud of its achievements to date. But more still is necessary'.

Part of this 'gear change' or 'necessary more' is the annual 30 hours of CPD, but like democracy and the pursuit of happiness, professional development is universally celebrated as something good, with little analysis of what it entails. Trorey (2002, 2; original emphasis) distinguishes between '*institutional development*' aimed at improving a whole organisation, often described as '*staff development*' and the more individual '*professional development*' involving 'pedagogic knowledge and subject expertise'. There is a difference in their primary instigation and CPD is normally under the control of the professional.

The voluminous *National Standards for Teaching and Supporting Learning in Further Education in England and Wales* were published by the Further Education National Training Organisation (FENTO) in 1999 as a statutory basis for teacher training qualifications in England and they included a commitment to 'engage in continuing professional development' (FENTO 1999, 23). Although significant within the initial training of teachers in FE, the so-called FENTO standards had little influence on practice (Nasta 2007). Three years later in 2002 the government published *Success for All: Reforming Further Education and Training – Our Vision for the Future*, which sought to put 'teaching, training and learning at the heart of what we do' (DfES 2002, 5). This highlighted CPD as a priority area because, in an astonishingly candid admission (DfES 2002, 4), 'insufficient attention [had] been given to improving teaching, training and learning'. It was, therefore, the aim of the government to: '...address under-investment in professionalism and to reward and recognise the importance of the further education and training workforce' (DfES 2002, 5).

As a part of the *Success for All* programme the DfES published *Equipping Our Teachers for the Future* (DfES 2004), which spawned the new statutory period of CPD and a corresponding rise in control and scrutiny. Crucially, teachers in FE now need to record their annual CPD in order to achieve and maintain the status of 'Qualified Teacher in Learning and Skills' (QTLS), which is their licence to practise. These workforce reforms were introduced and positioned to be indisputably positive. Mandatory CPD was about 'updating knowledge of the subject taught and developing teaching skills' of individual teachers (Department for Innovation, Universities and Skills [DIUS] 2008, 1). However, LLUK's (2008b, 14) research on CPD in the sector found a discrepancy in views between teachers and managers suggesting this stress on individual teachers entails responsibility without control. Their data indicated 59% of teachers strongly agreed that lack of time was a barrier to 'accessing CPD opportunities', against only 25% of senior managers. Likewise, 33% of teachers strongly agreed that cost was a barrier, against 11% of senior managers. Managers may be blaming teachers for lack of professional development while ignoring other structural obstacles. Moreover, the same research (LLUK 2008b, 15) found that even what influence teachers have over their CPD was weak and that CPD is melding with staff development instigated by the organisation (LLUK 2008b, 10). Institutional control of CPD is encouraged by one of the anticipated outcomes in the government's *Workforce Strategy Implementation Plan* (LLUK 2008d, 10):

> A culture of CPD is established within the Further Education sector focused on meeting learner needs at provider and individual level. Colleges and learning providers approach their own staff development in similar and flexible ways, as they would for a learner, employer or client. The confidence and capacity of the workforce in understanding and using technology to transform education and training will be a key element of this culture.

Here, CPD and staff development become interchangeable, predominantly about the needs of the organisation and beyond the control of the individual. Moreover, in the guidance to staff entering FE from other education sectors quoted previously, LLUK (2008c, 6) explicitly recommends CPD as a means of coping with FE's vicissitudes:

> If you previously taught in the schools sector, you might have assumed you had chosen a lifetime's career. For teachers in FE, the fluidity, complexity and rapidly changing priorities mean that continuity is much more uncertain. One crucial way that practitioners in FE can deal with this uncertainty is to be proactive about their professional development.

This is some distance from the stated purpose of 'updating knowledge of the subject taught and developing teaching skills'. Moreover, mandatory professional development suffers from appearing as yet another initiative, and even the government recognises the sheer amount of policy as an impediment to achieving progress in FE. The DIUS business plan for 2008–2009 includes eight strategic messages; 15 'key policy deliverables'; two public service agreements; and six Departmental Strategy Objectives. Little wonder, then, that one of the department's 'top seven corporate risks' is:

> Sector instability and Reform Overload in FE – that the key delivery partners become distracted from delivering 'business as usual' due to uncertainty over the future organisational shape of the sector, or as a result of the sheer scale of change. (DIUS 2008, 6)

By the government's own admission the quantity of reforms makes them less likely to succeed, which may lead to the need for more reforms. This dubious logic is a feature of the gap between policy and practice.

What impact has compulsory CPD had?

Having described the policy context I now turn to the functioning of the CPD reform. The implementation plan for the workforce strategy (LLUK 2008d, 5) states that 'milestones and outcomes should be measurable', but LLUK (2008b, 4) are aware of the difficulty of assessing what effect CPD has had on the sector and the 'urgent need to develop more precise instruments for impact management'.

The ambiguity of 'impact measurement' is evident in anticipated outcome 3.2 in the implementation plan for the FE workforce strategy (LLUK 2008d, 10):

> A workforce that provides the impetus for its own learning needs by taking action towards individual skills development. This outcome will be demonstrated by the enthusiasm of staff about the new CPD opportunities available and their keenness to adopt new technologies and engage in the latest training.

Yet, quantifying enthusiasm or keenness is difficult and so quantitative targets take precedence; employers had to ensure that each teacher in FE was registered with IfL by September 2008 and that he or she records 30 hours of CPD each year (LLUK 2008d, 6). Though these targets were designed as a lever for policy and to assess the change that policy had made, the small-scale exploratory research described at the beginning of this paper suggests that they have already 'become an end in themselves' (Steer et al. 2007, 177). The responses to questionnaires from the 29 staff with responsibility for CPD and staff development at 21 FE organisations suggest how a reform can achieve little of what it was designed for, in this case increased participation in CPD, but still apparently succeed.

Although many respondents acknowledged that the CPD initiative was still relatively new, none indicated that it had made a significant difference to practice in institutions over 12 months after its introduction, though it had been experienced in managerialist accountability. However, the limitations of managerialism are also apparent in these data. One respondent to the research reflected this by writing about the 'ethos of counting hours rather than IMPACT' (original capitalisation), another identified the problem as being: '…that the actual purpose of CPD seems to be lost and the amount of CPD completed is the most important issue i.e., "tick box mentality"'.

Several others used this motif of 'ticking boxes' to describe the effect of compulsory CPD in organisations, while another described how CPD was viewed as 'jumping through hoops' because of the need to maintain QTLS. Nevertheless, the government's goal of a culture of CPD was widely supported. The perceived barriers to the creation of this culture were mainly structural, above all, time pressures on already full workloads. Moreover, 13 identified what might be summarised as obstacles relating to the existing culture in colleges, which had not hitherto promoted CPD. One respondent used the term 'entrenched attitudes'. Nonetheless, there were many instances of organisations genuinely attempting to develop the professional practice of their staff; one college had produced pamphlets on good practice for teachers; one had produced guides to teaching resources; and another had increased the number of staff supported on HE qualifications. Furthermore, organisations were running mandatory training days to make up some proportion of the 30 hours and others were producing online CPD materials. However, the instigation for these activities came largely from the organisation rather than the individual, and almost all had been in place prior to the new CPD initiative. One respondent described the situation at an FE college: 'Still very much a staff development approach with compulsory sessions that ensure staff can use college systems and are familiar of [*sic*] policies, rather than meaningful CPD'.

Similarly, a college elsewhere had issued all staff with a substantial portfolio to facilitate reflection on and recording of CPD prior to the introduction of mandatory CPD, but had provided '*no introduction, no guidelines, no follow up*' (original emphases).

Also apparent was the high level of management preparation to ensure recording of the 30 hours of CPD and membership of IfL. Respondents from all but two of the 21 organisations could describe the systems in place to achieve the government's 'headline actions' (LLUK 2008d). One college had a 'master spreadsheet'; others used databases; and others had 'frameworks' in place. Respondents described mechanisms of compliance to verify achievement of targets systematically and quantitatively, even where there had been little new engagement in CPD. This is not deception; the targets have been achieved because college managers working within an audit culture have become adept at creating systems to 'evidence' target achievement. The symbiotic nature of the relationship between targets and systems suggests a mutually dependent ecology of performance indicators and systems to indicate performance. Thus performativity flourishes separate from professional practice.

Writing about English FE in the 1990s Gleeson and Shain (1999, 482) described 'strategic compliance' as 'a form of artful pragmatism reconciling professional and managerial interests', which they identified among managers and teachers in FE who were coping with rapid change. Strategic compliers retained a commitment to traditional professional and educational values but partially agreed to reforms in line with senior college management to create space for manoeuvre and so defend what they valued in their practice. Strategic compliers 'did not comply for the 'sake of their own skins' (Gleeson and Shain 1999, 460), but made decisions to conform or resist based upon the needs of their learners. Whether such space exists in FE today is moot, but this does not explain the institutional response to the CPD initiative because the compliance here is expedient not strategic. In other words, the mechanisms of compliance are pragmatic, but are not part of a strategy to defend educational values.

Colleges contend for government funding and managers must be seen to achieve targets because their institution depends on finance directly related to those targets. In this artificial market only financial messages are credible and this has created a democratic deficit where those affected by policy have little influence over it. Since college managers have little control over policy implementation and since the government's vision for FE appears unachievable, they will tell the government the 'truth', targets have been achieved; but not the whole 'truth', those targets do not reflect changed practice.

This picture of the early implementation of the CPD initiative illustrates the limitations of top-down, outcomes-led policymaking. It demonstrates how an initiative can appear successful without achieving the intended change in practice because colleges can report performance indicators have been met, even where few staff have heard of the reform. While the government's policy levers become apparently more numerous and rigorous, they are not as powerful as the government's rhetoric might suggest. The gap between policy and practice remains.

Conclusion

New Labour has invested more in FE in England than any previous government because they identified the sector as a vehicle to deliver their core policies of global competitiveness through a high-skills workforce and social justice through widening participation in education. The links between national economic competitiveness, social justice and education are currently hegemonic and central to New Labour orthodoxy, but these links remain unfounded and consequently FE can only fail to achieve the government's central goals. This failure has led to closer scrutiny and control of the sector and to so many policy initiatives that 'reform overload' is a risk recognised even by the government. Paradoxically those same initiatives may be reported as successful, even where little has changed. The trajectory of policy for CPD from voluntarism to statutory compulsion uncovers one instance of this process in action. In a symbiotic response to the government's requirement to measure impact through numerical targets, college managers have pragmatically constructed systems to report achievement of the numerical targets attached to CPD, despite insignificant alteration in patterns of practice. This symbiotic response derives from the unequal and undemocratic relationship between colleges and the government. This situation can only be ameliorated when those working and studying in colleges have more control over setting their own collective priorities, including CPD, in a rational rather than a performative manner.

References

Avis, J. 2003. Re-thinking trust in a performative culture: The case of education. *Journal of Education Policy* 8, no. 3: 315–32.

Avis, J. 2007. *Education, policy and social justice.* London: Continuum.

Ball, S. 1999. Labour, learning and the economy: A 'policy sociology' perspective. *Cambridge Journal of Education* 29, no. 2: 195–206.

Ball, S. 2008. *The education debate.* Bristol, UK: Policy Press.

Brown, P., H. Lauder, and D. Ashton. 2008. *Education, globalisation and the knowledge economy. A Commentary by the Teaching and Learning Research Programme.* London: TLRP.

Coffield, F. 1999. Breaking the consensus: Lifelong learning as social control. *British Educational Research Journal* 25, no. 4: 479–99.

Coffield, F., S. Edward, I. Finlay, A. Hodgson, K. Spours, and R. Steer. 2008. *Improving learning, skills and inclusion: The impact of policy on post-compulsory education.* Abingdon, UK: Routledge.

Coffield, F., S. Edward, I. Finlay, A. Hodgson, K. Spours, R. Steer, and M. Gregson. 2007. How policy impacts on practice and how practice does not impact on policy. *British Educational Research Journal* 33, no. 5: 723–41.

DfEE. 1998. *The learning age: Renaissance for a new Britain.* Green Paper Cmnd 3790. London: The Stationery Office.

DfEE. 1999. *Learning to succeed: A new framework for post-16 learning.* London: The Stationery Office.

DfES. 2002. *Success for all: Reforming further education and training.* London: The Stationery Office.

DfES. 2004. *Equipping our teachers for the future.* London: The Stationery Office.

DfES. 2006. *Further education: Raising skills, improving life chances.* London: The Stationery Office.

DIUS. 2008. *DIUS 2008–09 business plan at a glance: Investing in our future.* London: DIUS.

Finlay, I., K. Spours, R. Steer, F. Coffield, M. Gregson, and A. Hodgson. 2007. 'The heart of what we do': Policies on teaching, learning and assessment in the new learning and skills sector. *Journal of Vocational Education and Training* 59, no. 2: 137–54.

Foster, A. 2005. *Realising the potential: A review of the future role of further education colleges.* London: DfES.

FENTO. 1999. *National standards for teaching and supporting learning in further education in England and Wales.* London: FENTO.

Gleeson, D., and F. Shain. 1999. Managing ambiguity: Between markets and managerialism – a case study of middle managers in further education. *The Sociological Review* 47, no. 3: 461–90.

Hall, S. 2003. New Labour's double shuffle. *Soundings* 24. http://www.lwbooks.co.uk/journals/articles/nov03.html.

IfL. 2008. Sector acronyms and abbreviations. Institute for Learning. http://www.ifl.ac.uk/about-ifl/glossary/acronyms-and-abbreviations.

IfL. 2009. Licence to practise: Professional formation your guide to qualified teacher learning and skills (QTLS) and associate teacher learning and skills (ATLS) status. Institute for Learning. http://www.ifl.ac.uk/__data/assets/pdf_file/0019/4771/ProfessionalFormation Supportpackwebsite250209.pdf.

Kennedy, H. 1997. *Learning works: Widening participation in further education.* Coventry: FEFC.

Learning and Skills Council. 2005. *Learning and skills – the agenda for change: The Prospectus.* Coventry, UK: LSC.

Leitch, S. 2006. *Prosperity for all in the global economy: World class skills, final report.* London: The Stationery Office.

LLUK. 2006. *New overarching professional standards for teachers, tutors and trainers in the lifelong learning sector.* London: LLUK.

LLUK. 2008a. *Workforce strategy for the further education system in England, 2007–2012.* London: LLUK.

LLUK. 2008b. *Access to effective and equitable continuing professional development opportunities for teachers, tutors and trainers in the lifelong learning sector.* London: LLUK.

LLUK. 2008c. *Orientation guidance for qualified teachers entering further education.* London: LLUK.

LLUK. 2008d. *Workforce strategy for the further education sector in England 2007–2012: Implementation plan.* London: LLUK.

Lucas, N. 2004. The 'FENTO fandango': National standards, compulsory teaching qualifications and the growing regulation of FE college teachers. *Journal of Further and Higher Education* 28, no. 1: 35–51.

Morris, E. 2001. Professionalism and trust – the future of teachers and teaching. A speech by the secretary of state for education to the social market foundation, 12 November, in London.

Nasta, T. 2007. Translating national standards into practice for the initial teaching of Further Education (FE) teachers in England. *Research in Post-Compulsory Education* 12, no. 1: 1–17.

Orr, K. 2008. Room for improvement? The impact of compulsory professional development for teachers in England's further education sector. *Journal of In Service Education* 34, no. 1: 97–108.

Rikowski, G. 2001. Education for industry: A complex technicism. *Journal of Education and Work* 14: 29–49.

Steer, R., K. Spours, A. Hodgson, I. Finlay, F. Coffield, S. Edward, and M. Gregson. 2007. 'Modernisation' and the role of policy levers in the learning and skills sector. *Journal of Vocational Education and Training* 59, no. 2: 175–92.

Tomlinson, S. 2001. *Education in a post-welfare society.* Buckingham, UK: Open University Press.

Trorey, G. 2002. Introduction: Meeting the needs of the individual and the institution. In *Professional development and institutional needs,* ed. G. Trorey, and C. Cullingford, 1–14. Aldershot, UK: Ashgate.

One step forward, two steps back? The professionalisation of further education teachers in England

Norman Lucas

This paper draws upon two research projects to evaluate a decade of reform concerning the professionalisation of further education teachers, and discusses future prospects under the new coalition government. It suggests that policy initiatives to regulate further education (FE) teachers have taken place within an industrial or occupational paradigm of the past that keeps FE separate from the more professional frameworks of schools and higher education. Drawing upon research, the paper also shows that after a decade of reform, successive standards and regulatory frameworks have not brought about national coherence. Rather, it has fragmented the system even further and diverted attention away from addressing more fundamental weaknesses such as developing stronger mentoring and workplace support. In conclusion, the analysis looks to the future, arguing that the threatened revocation of the 2007 regulations, combined with the present economic situation facing colleges, will lead to the marketisation of FE initial teacher training. This has profound implications for the quality of provision and the professional status of FE teachers, who seem to be returning to their voluntarist past.

A decade of reform under New Labour: from neglect to regulation

Unlike schools, until the late 1990s, the training of teachers in further and adult education (FE) in England had been the subject of little regulation by government. There had been changes in the governance and funding of FE colleges in the previous decade (Lucas 2004) but not the professional training of FE teachers. Teacher education in FE was mostly in-service, *ad hoc* and uneven. This system was largely voluntarist, with initial training and staff development dependent on the attitudes of college employers. Professional training tended to be haphazard, reflecting the diverse nature of FE and the marginalisation of vocational and technical education (Robson 1998).

In 1997, the New Labour government announced their concern about raising teaching standards in FE as colleges became central to the government's plans to improve skills as an important ingredient in boosting the economy and enhancing national competitiveness (Orr 2009). As FE moved up the political agenda so the sector itself and its teachers became subject to greater state regulation. In 1997 the government announced its intention of introducing a requirement for all new FE teachers to have a teaching qualification based upon national standards. In 1999, a new employer-led body, the Further Education National Training Organisation (FENTO), published national standards for FE teachers (FENTO 1999) and two years later a new statutory instrument was introduced by the Department for Education and Skills (DfES) giving legislative authority for the new initial teacher training (ITT) regime (DfES 2001). Further standards and requirements were introduced for teachers of adult basic skills (DfES 2002) and the government monitored the operation of the new system through the publication of targets for teacher education (DfES 2004).

No sooner had the reforms been introduced than a major national survey inspection of FE teacher education by Her Majesty's Inspectorate (HMI) (Ofsted 2003) reached the damning conclusion that the existing system, based on the FENTO standards, provided an unsatisfactory foundation for the professional development of FE teachers at the start of their careers. The survey identified a huge variability in the quality of teacher training, painting a stark picture of inadequate support and opportunities for trainees to develop their specialist teaching skills.

These weaknesses were linked to a lack of subject mentoring in the workplace and insufficient observations and feedback on trainees' teaching practice. Often trainees were found to have a very narrow professional experience of education and training. For example, they lacked opportunities for teaching and assessing students of different types, at different levels and in different institutions. Her Majesty's Inspectorate reported that the taught elements of ITT courses were generally good yet there were too few connections made between the taught elements of the course and the supervision and assessment of a trainee's teaching in the workplace. The government of the time reacted swiftly to this criticism. A policy document, *Equipping our Teachers for the Future* (DfES 2004), was published that purported to offer a solution to the problems identified by HMI. It committed the government to an ambitious set of reforms, including new regulations and standards, by September 2007. The Further Education National Training Organisation was abolished in 2005 and replaced by a new employer-led body, the sector skills council Lifelong Learning UK (LLUK). The FENTO standards were replaced by new national standards, role specifications and learning outcomes (LLUK 2007). The overall aim of government policy was to create a national system for further education ITT qualifications comparable to that operating in the schools sector that would raise the professional status of teachers in post-compulsory education. Lifelong Learning UK attempted to introduce a more standardised approach by supplementing the new national standards with core units of assessment based on an agreed credit framework. This was intended to enable trainees to transfer between different institutions during their training. The government was also keen to overcome the gap between what was taught on the course and what happened in the workplace, to develop a more subject specialist approach to ITT and, in particular, to provide better specialist mentoring support in the workplace.

The new qualifications structure comprised three qualifications: an initial ITT qualification, Preparing to Teach in the Lifelong Learning Sector (PTLLS), the Certificate in Teaching in the Lifelong Learning Sector (CTLLS) and the Diploma in Teaching in the Lifelong Learning Sector (DTLLS). The CTLLS was designed for a category of teachers, known as associate teachers, seen as having a narrower role in the design of curricula, teaching materials and assessment. The DTLLS was for full or part-time teachers and other staff with wide responsibilities for teaching, managing courses and supporting students. All these qualifications were planned to be compatible within a national credit framework to reflect the distinction between full-teacher and associate-teacher roles (Thompson and Robinson 2008). This new system was highly prescriptive: each qualification had to incorporate not just the LLUK standards, but also LLUK units of assessment that specified the learning outcomes and assessment criteria (LLUK 2007). In addition, all higher education institutions (HEIs) had to have their ITT programmes endorsed by Standards Verification UK (SVUK), a subsidiary of LLUK, until March 2011, and were subject to annual monitoring by SVUK.

In their requirements, LLUK stressed the importance for ITT courses to provide subject mentors in the workplace – all trainees on DTLLS or equivalent courses would be required to have eight observations of their teaching practice, of which at least four would be observed by their specialist mentors. A new professional status, Qualified Teacher Learning and Skills (QTLS), comparable to Qualified Teacher Status for school teachers, was also introduced. Once FE trainees had completed their initial training, they would be required to embark on a period of 'professional formation' in order to gain QTLS and become 'fully' qualified. However, unlike in the schools sector, QTLS is subject to a post-qualification period where teachers have to provide evidence of engaging in 30 hours of continuous professional development (CPD) per annum and demonstrate a minimum of a level-two standard in literacy and numeracy. Unlike the school sector, where there is an obligation under newly qualified teacher status for the school itself to take responsibility, the onus for gaining QTLS is on the individual FE teacher. Qualified Teacher Learning and Skills must be completed within five years and is awarded by the Institute for Learning (IfL), a body re-designed and launched in 2007 to grant QTLS and to raise the professional standing of FE teachers. The QTLS is then subject to annual renewal based upon evidence of appropriate CPD by the individual teacher. Those with CTLLS who were associate teachers could apply for a lesser status: Associate Teacher Learning and Skills. Very little support accompanied the reforms to address the systemic weaknesses in college workplaces identified by the 2003 HMI survey. Improving workplace practice was to be addressed through the creation of Centres for Excellence in Teacher Training (CETTs), regionally based partnerships that were expected to foster good practice amongst providers. The CETTS were allocated £30 million for three years, after which time they were expected to become self-financing. This amount spread over the entire 'learning and skills sector' represented a relatively small resource.

Professionalism and the industrial paradigm of FE reform

As shown below, the reform process concerning the professionalisation and regulation of teachers in further education has followed a unique trajectory: Table 1.

The state regulation in the form of standards to professionals in schools, FE and higher education (HE) all represent efforts by the State to regulate professional practice. However, as Lucas and Nasta (2010) argue, the form they take and the wider context in which they have been applied have been poles apart, with a quite different emphasis on how standards should be applied. In other studies, Raffe et al. (1997) and Bailey and Robson (2002) highlight the separate traditions of training school, college and HE teachers, arguing that the separation appears to be as strong as ever,

Table 1.   Labour reform of FE teacher training: a timeline.

- 1997–1999: DfES consultation on introduction of standards and qualifications for FE teachers
- 1999: Formation of FENTO and publication of the national occupational standards
- 2001: Statutory instrument
    – New teachers required to gain a teaching qualification based upon approved national standards (FENTO)
    – Ofsted given responsibility for inspection
- 2002: Subject specifications for teachers of adult literacy, numeracy and ESOL
- 2003: Publication of the critical HMI national survey on the initial training of FE teachers and DfES consultation on future reforms
- 2004: Publication by DfES of *Equipping our Teachers for the Future* – reforming initial teacher training for the learning and skills sector
- 2005: DfES pilots – subject mentoring, observation of teaching practice and so on. The LLUK and SVUK replace FENTO
- 2006: Publication of LLUK standards for teachers in the learning and skills sector. Publication of draft criteria for the award of CETT status. Publication by DfES of *Professionalisation of the Learning and Skills Sector* announcing plans for a compulsory CPD requirement for FE teachers
- 2007: Publication of LLUK mandatory units of assessment for ITT (England). Regulations introduced by DIUS (Department for Innovation, Universities and Skills) introducing QTLS and a compulsory CPD requirement. First member joins professional body the Institute for Learning (IfL)
- 2008: Implementation of reforms – ITT providers go through SVUK endorsement and commence teaching and assessing ITT qualifications based upon the new LLUK standards and assessment units. (based upon Lucas, Nasta, and Rogers 2012)

as is a trend of ever greater and more complex forms of regulation. Drawing from this, Lucas and Nasta suggest that much like our qualifications system the regulation of professionals in school, HE and FE can be seen as occupying three different and distinct tracks because of the origin of the regulations, what happened to them en-route and the contexts to which they were applied.

For example, in HE there is no regulatory framework and the permissive nature of the professional standards allows institutions to create their own curricula. The standards applied to schools, while prescriptive, are in their third iteration, having been mediated by school-teachers and university providers of ITT courses to provide a framework or 'common understanding' that stresses the importance of professional judgment made at different times and in different contexts. Unlike schools and HE teachers, FE teachers are treated differently because they are essentially locked into an industrial or occupational model, as illustrated by the very different regulatory bodies: the Teacher Development Agency, a non-departmental government body; the Higher Education Academy, a limited company controlled by HE; and the employer-led Sector Skills Council, LLUK. Further Education alone has an employer-led body yet, as suggested above, ITT and QTLS fall on the individual not the employer. This industrial tradition has powerful historical roots and has influenced the culture of FE itself.

In their analysis, Lucas and Nasta (2010) suggest that the inadequacy of the FENTO standards was challenged not by FE professionals or college employers but by an Office for Standards in Education (Ofsted) report (2003). The report found the standards inadequate and suggested that FE teachers should be placed within a framework more akin to that of schoolteachers. Instead, the DfES (2004), continuing the industrial paradigm, put in place a new framework with new standards based essentially on an occupational framework policed by an employer-led sector-skills council, the LLUK. They designed a new set of qualification guidelines with standards and units of assessment containing prescribed learning outcomes and assessment criteria that are 'mapped' against ITE courses.

Thus, a focus on the different cultures and traditions in schools, FE colleges and universities has a marked influence on the origin of professional standards and how they are used. Each transition entails processes of mediation and a re-contextualisation of knowledge. The intrinsic problem to do with the nature of the codified knowledge that standards represent is that the whole basis of standards-led reform of professionalism can be seen as fundamentally ill-conceived unless standards are viewed as something that is necessarily transformed when applied to different circumstances and contexts.

This is not to suggest that standards cannot be useful if used as a guide, allowing for professional interpretation according to different contexts, and to recognise that, like all cultural tools, they are transformed through mediation. They are not simply transferred from the policy to the pedagogical context, even when more and more specifications are added (Lucas and Nasta 2009). However, such a position is a very different perspective from those of policy makers in the government and regulatory bodies, who view standards as unambiguous outcomes, externally supplied curricular commodities that can be translated into professional practice.

In other words, as standards move between different contexts they are interpreted and used in very different ways. The role of the state (Secretary of State) and its agencies as 'producers' of standards is always mediated by the other agencies that are involved and most critically by the workplace environments where teacher-educators and trainees have to turn them into curricula and training programmes. The consequence of taking this theoretical position is that standards are not neutral because they embody assumptions about the nature of professionalism, qualifications and knowledge reflecting the relationships of power and authority and the cultural norms in different institutional and subject settings (Lucas and Nasta 2009). Focusing on mediation in this context raises issues about how standards are interpreted and used by the subjects for whom they were ostensibly designed. In such a situation, the power of professional identity and organisation has an influence on how standards are actually used. For example, the influence of school and HE professionals has been far more effective than that of the fragmented and impoverished professionalism in FE colleges.

In the context of further education teachers, the 192 professional standards are not left at the level of statements, they are broken down to smaller specifications and performance criteria (outcomes) – very much like the work-based National Vocational Qualification, which can then be used to assess trainees. The problem with this sort of approach is that when national standards (or any other prescriptive code) leave government and national agencies, they are interpreted in many different ways, not always leading to a commonality of practice and often having quite unintended consequences (Lucas and Nasta 2009). There are no standards for measuring standards so in order to apply standards across many contexts, regulatory bodies revert to the deceptive certainty of technicist models and to the comfort zone of further detailed statement specifications and competency statements and specifications, which in turn become new travelling artefacts.

The failure of FE teachers in the last decade to make the transition from an occupational/industrial to a professional track similar to school and HE professionals is complex and has not just been imposed through state regulation. One factor has been the relative weakness of intermediary bodies such as employer organisations, trade unions and professional organisations in FE that could have mediated the standards. Another lies in senior college managers and FE teachers themselves, many of whom have been reluctant to be identified with school-teachers and have defended their industrial past and differences with other sectors of education (Lucas 2004). Divisions also exist between large FE colleges, adult providers and sixth form colleges. This in turn reflects the diversity of FE and the tensions between different subject and vocational specialisms and the divisions between the significant numbers of full-time and part-time teaching staff. Furthermore, all recent policy initiatives to regulate FE teachers have taken place within a fragmented and impoverished professional culture, which often has a weak work-based culture of supporting trainees and the professional development of its teachers (Lucas and Unwin 2009). In such a context, the industrial or occupational paradigm of the past keeps the FE teachers separate from the more professional framework of others in schools and HE.

An assessment: the gap between policy intention and actual outcomes

As suggested above, the aim of government policy was the application of new national standards in order to create a national system for ITT qualifications to enable trainees to transfer between different institutions during their training. Alongside this, the QTLS framework, including compulsory CPD, would raise the professional status of FE teachers. The broad policy intention to improve the quality of teacher training was to overcome the gap between what was taught on the course and what happened in the workplace. The focus was upon developing a more subject-specialist approach to ITT and, in particular, to provide better specialist mentoring in the workplace.

Recent research among HEIs (Lucas, Nasta, and Rogers 2012) indicates that the complex regulatory framework put in place based upon statutory regulation, standards and assessment units has not led to what policy makers intended. The evidence in Figure 1 shows that HEIs are offering qualifications at different levels with different names and carrying different volumes of academic credit. For example, DTLLS was offered at levels 4 and 5, a Certificate of Education (Cert Ed) at levels 4, 5 and 6 and a Post-Graduate Certificate of Education (PGCE) at level 7 (Masters Level). Credits ranged from 6 to 30 per module. Put together, this makes the policy aim of allowing learners to transfer modules between universities seem impossible. The research evidence suggests that the creation of a national ITT system regulated by LLUK and SVUK has not led to greater consistency or standardisation, leading to confusion among teachers and managers.

Evidence also pointed to the difficulties teacher-educators have experienced in providing adequate support for trainees to develop skills in teaching their specialist area. The research found HEIs unable to meet the wide specialist areas offered in FE colleges. As a consequence, trainees were primarily dependent upon the support of specialist mentors, who observed them teaching and gave wider guidance about specialist qualifications and assessment.

From interviews and focus groups there was general agreement that subject mentoring was still very uneven, with college management not able to provide the

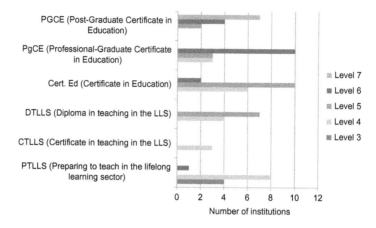

Figure 1.   Levels and names of awards offered by higher education institutions.
Source: Lucas, Nasta, and Rogers (2012).

resources to support systematic mentoring of trainees. All respondents agreed that the vast majority of work-based mentors had insufficient time to become familiar with the details of the ITT courses and were unable to help trainees make connections between what was taught and what happened in practice. Only 10% of those surveyed offered some sort of module choice that allowed trainees to develop skills related to their subject, for example in construction or engineering, or teaching context, such as adult and community learning or prison education. For the remaining 90%, it was reported that skills related to specialist teaching were 'embedded' within the modules offered, where trainees were encouraged to explore questions through their subject or vocational specialism. The reality seemed to be that there is little, if any, choice of specialist modules from the perspective of the trainee because of costs and logistics.

With the exception of Skills for Life ITT courses, which do require subject specialist options and qualifications, the survey found no specific options concerning subject specialism or areas such as 14–19 education and training, vocational learning, adult learning, specific learning difficulties and disabilities, or prison education. Overall, it seemed that despite the rhetoric of the reform, the sheer diversity of FE and adult provision linked to finite resources made it very difficult within the ITT course to provide option modules. Furthermore, the award designed for those in associate teaching roles, CTTLS, has had limited take-up. Specialist options are rarely available and support for trainees to develop their specialist teaching skills remains weak. The holistic process of developing as a teacher may be reduced to a fragmented approach of ticking boxes to fulfil LLUK assessment criteria. The system was described by one interviewee as a 'national shambles'. Of the responses from HEIs to an open-ended question about the advantages and disadvantages of the new regulatory regime, 90% were towards the negative. The government aim of professionalising the role of the FE teacher through the introduction of QTLS is not widely understood by college managers.

The policy aim of improving mentoring in the workplace has also been researched by Lucas and Unwin (2009). This work was carried out among a range of vocational and general teachers undergoing in-service teacher training in FE colleges. The result of the research revealed a picture of the ways in which the demands and pressures that shape the everyday workplace in FE colleges restrict the capacity of trainee teachers to learn and develop their professional expertise at work and also to build on their off-the-job learning. From the research, a number of themes emerged.

The first theme was the lack of support given to the trainee in the workplace. For example, only 10% were receiving any remission from their contracted hours to study for their teacher training courses over and above attending the mandatory taught sessions. The majority spoke about how they had struggled to balance their college workload with their studies. This was particularly the case with vocational teachers who struggle with the academic requirements of the assessed part of the course. The research showed that colleges did not respect the important principle of bestowing on trainees the dual identity of learner (trainee) and worker (teacher), with all that entails in providing practical support to trainees from more experienced colleagues and a reduced teaching load to provide time for trainees to benefit from off-the-job learning and to reflect upon and experiment with their learning (Fuller and Unwin 2004a). The teachers themselves regarded this state of affairs as a simple fact of life and the initial teaching qualifications and professional development of teachers relied on the goodwill and determination of the teachers themselves in the face of little support from elsewhere. The new requirement for FE teachers to acquire their 'licence to practice' has not really changed the culture within colleges.

The research also highlighted how teachers learnt in the workplace through informal learning and sharing of expertise as part of everyday practice. This theme emerged because part of the research project asked teachers to keep 'learning logs' (Fuller and Unwin 2004b) for a number of weeks to provide a record of how and what trainee teachers learn within the workplace. None of the logs recorded a learning encounter with their mentor. This is particularly significant because the teacher training reforms described above rely on mentors to give subject specialist support. This is a fundamental outcome of the 2007 reforms. The data showed that whilst the majority of trainee teachers had been allocated a mentor, they rarely had contact with them and learnt in more informal ways within departments with other colleagues. There was evidence of some good intentions on the part of managers and mentors but these often did not materialise because of the struggle to find time and space. Effectively, this sometimes resulted in trainee teachers getting no subject-specialist mentoring. Typically, the community of practice of teachers in FE is fragmented and fluid, dissolving and then reforming throughout the day. Putting all these factors together illustrates how difficult it is to provide consistent and reliable support for trainee teachers in the college workplace. Finding dedicated mentors with enough time to devote to the development of trainees' subject pedagogy is the exception rather than the norm.

The last theme that became apparent from the research was the separation of the ITT from the CPD and organisational strategy of the colleges. The mandatory requirement for all vocational or general college teachers in England to acquire a teaching qualification and to undergo 30 hours of CPD for a full-time teacher (pro-rata for part-time) means that, regardless of the length of their actual teaching experience, they participate in a form of apprenticeship. It was apparent from the research that initial training provision in most colleges is very much conceived of and practised as a tightly bounded process that is completely separate from colleges' CPD programmes or workforce development provision more generally. Furthermore, Lucas and Unwin (2009) argue that in many colleges the FE workplace remains an actual barrier to professional development, despite all the recent specifications and regulations.

The general tenor of the findings discussed above is echoed in other official reports on the FE sector. A recent Ofsted (2010) report highlighted that three quarters of providers were not aware of QTLS, four fifths made little progress in ensuring that all teachers met minimum levels of literacy and numeracy and there was 'considerable confusion about how to interpret the details of the reforms' (4). The report of the Skills Commission (2009) draws attention to the unsatisfactory state of the training of vocational teachers, which has often been a 'second thought' for policy makers and been 'relegated to the second division of teaching'. The Commission argues strongly for convergence between the separate training routes and regulatory structures of school, FE and HE teachers in FE, so that teachers across the sectors can work successfully across the 14–19 phase.

From the research available, the aim of creating a coherent national system of ITT must be seen as a failure. It is difficult, however, to assess if there has been progress in the quality of initial training and CPD of FE teachers. The introduction of compulsory teacher training and CPD is broadly supported by the FE sector. Yet Orr (2009) shows that college managers have constructed systems to report and show that numerical targets have been achieved but little has changed in terms of the impact on patterns and quality of CPD because the whole exercise has been one of 'ticking boxes' and 'counting hours' rather than focusing on the purpose and impact of CPD. Furthermore, Ofsted (2011) in their annual report show that teaching standards have deteriorated in colleges. The cause of this could be one of many things, such as cuts in funding and the employment of more part-time or unqualified staff. For example, Broad (2010) estimated in a FE workforce survey that 20% were agency staff. As far as ITE is concerned, there is evidence that the number of trainees is declining in some areas and that some providers are taking on unqualified staff who find it difficult to meet the entry requirements of ITT courses (LLUK 2010). These teachers are covered by the five-year period to gain teaching qualifications so they can continue for at least that long. This is not to say that FE teacher training is in some sort of crisis. It has always been challenged to meet the diverse needs of its teachers, and part-time teachers have always been a part of the landscape. The point is that despite a decade of reform, many of the problems discussed above, which are endemic to the sector, still remain.

It is hard to escape the conclusion that after a decade of reform, successive standards and regulatory frameworks have not brought about national coherence and, in many respects, have fragmented the system even further. The overwhelming message from those who have had to design ITT programmes in response to quickly changing standards and assessment requirements is that being forced to play a game of complying with external standards and regulations has diverted attention from addressing more fundamental weaknesses, such as developing stronger mentoring and workplace support and achieving a better synergy between the taught and practice elements of courses. The systemic weaknesses identified in the HMI survey in 2003 have not been successfully addressed.

The future: a step forward or back?

The election of a new government in May 2010 put many of the reforms of the last decade 'on hold'. This was because of the pledge to massively cut public expenditure and have a 'bonfire of Quangos'. Along with other Quangos, the cuts led to the abolition of, or 'de-licencing' of, LLUK and SVUK in 2011. Their functions were formally transferred to the Learning and Skills Improvement Service (LSIS) and the IfL. In practice, the absence of a sector skills council has left the LLUK standards in limbo. With no extra resources, the IfL has undertaken the work of SVUK in endorsing qualifications. Anecdotal evidence suggests that the IfL is simply not able to carry through the SVUK endorsement process and ITT courses are approved 'on the nod' if they have been through the awarding bodies' own quality assurance procedures. The irony is that although the intention of the government was to cut public expenditure, the abolition of LLUK and SVUK could be seen as an advance to the absurd 'mapping fandango' of the past to get endorsement, which, as the research shows, has not led to the intended improvements or national coherence.

An important document to note for the future is *New Challenges, New Chances. Further Education and Skills System Reform Plan: Building a World-Class Skills System* (BIS 2011). As the title indicates, much like the policy of the last government, FE is put at the centre of the strategy to raise skills as an essential part of economic growth. In order to reach 'world class skills' the document says it is necessary to pursue excellence in teaching and learning. It states that while there is good teaching in colleges, the latest annual inspection report (Ofsted 2011) found too little outstanding and good teaching. Some of the phrases used in the document, such as 'ensure there is a clear sector owned policy to support outstanding teaching and learning' (16), remain ambiguous, while there are clear proposals to establish independent commissions. This includes adult education and vocational teaching and learning, focusing on STEM (Science, Technology, Engineering and Mathematics) subjects. The report proposes three further actions. Firstly, to set up a review of professionalism in the FE and skills sector. Secondly, to set up a bursary development fund to explore new models of delivering initial teacher education. And, thirdly, to build a network of expert practitioners in specific vocational skills. This will 'build excellence in dual professionalism in key industry areas, and will also contribute to the expert training for annual UK skills competitions and international competitions' (BIS 2011, 17). All of the proposals will be implemented through LSIS.

The 'independent' review of professionalism in the further education and skills sector has got underway and has published its interim report (BIS 2012b). The term 'independent' is open to question as the commission is led by Lord Lichfield, who was formally Sir Bob Balchin, head of the grant maintained schools trust under the Thatcher Government (Noble-Rogers 2012). The commission's terms of reference are to review and examine the appropriateness of current regulation arising from 'Equipping out Teachers', discussed above, to raise professional standards and status of the FE and skills workforce and examine the role and future of the IfL and to consider the best way of facilitating a professionalised workforce in the FE and skills sector.

At the time of writing, the interim report of the review of professionalism in further education was published (BIS 2012b) and out for consultation. If the recommendations are implemented, they will have a profound effect on teacher qualifications and training. On the one hand, the recommendations include the proposal that Ofsted should look at an employer's commitment to the training and development of its workforce, the abolition of the Associate Teacher role and a review of teacher qualifications, much of which is suggested by the research discussed above. On the other hand, it states that 'we emphasise our core belief that staff training, professional updating, competency and behaviour are essentially matters between employers and employees' (6). The commission recommends the revocation of the 2007 Regulations from 1 September 2012, with 'largely discretionary advice to employers on appropriate qualifications for staff and continuous professional development replacing compulsion' (5). In other words, the end of regulations making a teaching qualification compulsory within the FE sector.

The review also confirms the end during 2012–2013 to State funding to the IfL, with support for professionalism among FE staff to be provided from September 2012 by the LSIS. Concerns have been widely expressed about the IfL's role, its 'value for money' and power as well as its reluctance to introduce a code of ethics, rather than a code of conduct, based upon employer needs (Plowright and Barr 2012). The unpopularity of the IfL among FE teachers, the removal of compulsory registration and professional formation recommended by the commission make the IfL's future precarious. In effect, if the recommendations are accepted, QTLS seems doomed, and the IfL with it. This is particularly problematic as the government has accepted the recommendations of the Wolf report (2011). This recommends that teachers with QTLS status should be allowed to teach in schools. Evidence suggests that the barriers preventing FE teachers from going into school are soon to be removed following consultation (UCET 2011). The implications and details of the change have yet to be thought through and the problems become particularly acute in the light of the commission's recommendations.

Whether the commission's recommendations are implemented remains to be seen. The implications are enormous for the professionalisation of FE teachers. However, all the policy initiatives and future development of professionalism in the FE sector need to be understood against the general economic context of cuts in public expenditure and, in particular, the cuts in FE. It is estimated that 2012 will see cuts of as much as 12% (Exley 2012), to say nothing of the implication of the introduction of loans for over 25-year-old learners in 2013. The FE sector is facing hard times and there is already evidence of colleges withdrawing budgets for teacher education and professional development (BIS 2012a). This does not bode well for the proposal to leave professional qualifications to employers.

The issue concerning ITT provision is also one of concern as cost is passed to the learner. The new bursaries for FE teachers of £1000 available for half of the 20,000 ITT teachers each year put financial pressure on FE teachers, particularly part-time teachers. The position is particularly stark when compared with bursaries of between £5000 and £20,000 for school-teacher ITT (Exley 2012). The average tuition fees for FE ITT courses in universities are set to rise to £9000 per year or £4500 for a two-year part-time course. Even if the cost is cut somewhat, university FE ITT courses will become very expensive and non-viable. Colleges can insist on staff attending cheaper in-house provision and private providers can offer this even more cheaply. For example, the Advanced Training Academy UK, a private Edexcel-approved provider, offers DTLLS on-line at a cost of £1500. The full teaching qualification can be achieved within six months and the entry requirement is a PTLLS qualification (offered in four days at a cost of £249.99) or a GCSE grade C or above (http//www.advancetraininguk.com). How such provision can be matched to school sector PGCEs is difficult to work out.

The revocation of the 2007 regulations (if it happens), the present economic situation facing colleges and the exit of universities and marketisation of FE ITT provision have profound implications for the quality of provision and, indeed, the professional status of FE teachers. It would seem that FE teachers are returning to their voluntarist past.

References

Bailey, B., and J. Robson. 2002. "Changing Teachers: A Critical Review of Recent Policies Affecting the Professional Training and Qualifications of Teachers in Schools, Colleges and Universities in England." *Journal of Vocational Education and Training* 54 (3): 325–342.

BIS. 2011. *New Challenges, New Chances. Further Education and Skills System Reform Plan; Building a World Class Skills System*. London: Department for Business, Innovation and Skills.

BIS. 2012a. *Evaluation of FE Teachers' Qualifications (England) Regulations 2007*. BIS Research Paper 66. London: Department for Business, Innovation and Skills.

BIS. 2012b. *Professionalism in Further Education*. Interim Report of the Independent Review Panel. London: Department for Business, Innovation and Skills.

Broad, J. 2010. "Organisational Approaches to the 'Professionalisation' Agenda: Planning the Provision of the New ITE Qualifications for the FE Sector." http//eprints.hud.ac.uk/11095

DfES (Department for Education and Skills). 2001. *The Post-16 Education and Training Inspection Regulations*. Statutory Instrument 2001 No. 799. London: Department of Education and Skills.

DfES (Department for Education and Skills). 2002. *Subject Specifications for Teachers of Adult Literacy and Numeracy*. London: DfES and FENTO.

DfES (Department for Education and Skills). 2004. *Equipping Our Teachers for the Future: Reforming Initial Teacher Training for the Learning and Skills Sector*. London: Department for Education and Skills, Standards Unit.

Exley, S. 2012. "New Bursaries Won't Sweeten the Pill of Tuition Fees." FE news. *Times Education Supplement,* March 2. http://www.tes.co.uk/article.aspx?storycode=6187376

FENTO (Further Education National Training Organisation). 1999. *National Standards for Teaching and Supporting Learning in Further Education in England and Wales*. London: FENTO.

Fuller, A., and L. Unwin. 2004a. "Expansive Learning Environments: Integrating Organisational and Personal Development." In *Workplace Learning in Context*, edited by L. Rainbird, A. Fuller, and A. Munro, 126–144. London: Routledge.

Fuller, A., and L. Unwin. 2004b. "Young People as Teachers and Learners in the Workplace: Challenging the Novice-Expert Dichotomy." *International Journal of Training and Development* 8 (1): 31–41.

LLUK (Lifelong Learning UK). 2007. *Developing Qualifications for Teachers, Tutors and Trainers in the Lifelong Learning Sector in England: Interim Information for Awarding Institutions*. London: Lifelong Learning UK.

LLUK (Lifelong Learning UK). 2010. *Recent Trend in the Initial Training of Teachers of Literacy Numeracy and ESOL for the Further Education Sector in England*. London: Lifelong Learning UK.

Lucas, N. 2004. *Teaching in Further Education: New Perspectives for a Changing Context*. Bedford Way Paper. London: Institute of Education, University of London.

Lucas, N., and T. Nasta. 2009. "How Standards Travel and Change between Contexts. National Standards for TVET Teacher Education in the UK. A Cautionary Tale." In *Standardisation in TVET Teacher Education*, edited by J. Diterich, J. Yunos, G. Spottl, and M. Bukit, 61–81. Frankfurt: Peter Lang.

Lucas, N., and T. Nasta. 2010. "State Regulation and the Professionalisation of Further Education Teachers: A Comparison with Schools and HE." *Journal of Vocational Education and Training* 62 (4): 441–454.

Lucas, N., T. Nasta, and L. Rogers. 2012. "From Fragmentation to Chaos? The Regulation of Initial Teacher Training in Further Education." *British Education Research Journal* 38 (4): 677–695.

Lucas, N., and L. Unwin. 2009. "Developing Teacher Expertise at Work: In-Service Trainee Teachers in Colleges of Further Education in England." *Journal of Further and Higher Education* 33 (4): 423–433.

Noble-Rogers, J. 2012. Speech given at ATL conference FE zone, Manchester, April 13.

OFSTED (Office for Standards in Education). 2003. *The Initial Training of Further Education Teachers: A Survey.* HMI 1762. London: OFSTED.

OFSTED (Office for Standards in Education). 2010. *Progress in Implementing Reforms in the Accreditation and Continuing Professional Development of Teachers in Further Education.* London: OFSTED.

OFSTED (Office for Standards in Education). 2011. *The Annual Report of Her Majesty's Chief Inspector of Education, Children's Services and Skills 2010/11.* London: OFSTED.

Orr, K. 2009. "Performativity and Professional Development: The Gap between Policy and Practice in the English Further Education Sector." *Research in Post-Compulsory Education* 14 (4): 478–489.

Plowright, D., and G. Barr. 2012. "An Integrated Professionalism in Further Education: A Time for Phronesis?" *Journal of Further and Higher Education* 36 (1): 1–16.

Raffe, D., K. Spours, M. Young, and C. Howieson. 1997. *The Unification of Post-Compulsory Education: Towards a Conceptual Framework.* London: Economic and Social Research Council.

Robson, J. 1998. "A Profession in Crisis: Status, Culture and Identity in the Further Education College." *Journal of Vocational Education and Training* 50 (4): 585–607.

Skills Commission. 2009. "Teacher Training in Vocational Education." Accessed October 29, 2010. www.policyconnect.org.uk

Thompson, R., and D. Robinson. 2008. "Changing Step or Marking Time? Teacher Education Reforms for the Learning and Skills Sector in England." *Journal of Further and Higher Education* 32 (2): 161–173.

UCET (Universities' Council for the Education of Teachers). 2011. "Consultation Response to DfE Consultation. 'Proposed Changes to Allow Qualified Teachers from Further Education and from the United States, Canada, Australia and New Zealand to Become Permanent Teachers in English Schools'." http://www.ucet.ac.uk/

Wolf Report. 2011. *Review of Vocational Education.* London: DfE.

Professional versus occupational models of work competence

Stan Lester

In addition to the familiar occupational standards that underpin National Vocational Qualifications, the UK has a parallel if less complete system of competence or practice standards that are developed and controlled by professional bodies. While there is a certain amount of overlap between the two types of standard, recent research points to a distinct professional, as opposed to occupational, perspective on work competence. This can be characterised as focusing on ethics, professionalism and key standards rather than the detail of roles and functions; being designed to apply across the profession rather than having a core-and-options structure; and providing confidence in practitioners' abilities to act as a member of the profession rather than in a bounded occupational role. These factors are illustrated by reference to practices in professions with which the author has worked, suggesting that there is a spectrum of approaches from this archetypally professional one to a more utilitarian, occupationally oriented one.

Introduction

Over the last 25 years, the United Kingdom (UK) has developed an aspirationally comprehensive system of setting role descriptions and standards of competence for work occupations. This system of national occupational standards is best known for underpinning National Vocational Qualifications (NVQs), and it continues to be used as the basis for many qualifications in the Qualifications and Credit Framework and in the separate Scottish system. Occupational standards follow a broadly common approach which assumes that all work can be expressed in terms of roles and functions and that these can be specified in more-or-less finite terms. They were originally introduced as part of a policy reform designed to improve the relevance of vocational education and training, and not least to provide meaningful qualifications for young people on government-funded training programmes; initially focusing on less complex kinds of work, they were quickly extended to management and now include many occupations that typically involve graduate or postgraduate entry. Most occupational standards are now developed and managed by Sector Skills Councils (SSCs), government-endorsed and at least nominally employer-led bodies that can generally trace their origins back to the NVQ lead bodies of two decades ago, and in some cases to the industry training boards set up in the 1960s.

The UK also has a long-established and influential (if more loosely defined) system of professions, working principally at what might be termed the upper end of the education and training spectrum. Professions have generally been responsible for the standards of education, practice and conduct of their members, archetypally through regulatory bodies or self-governing associations that set, monitor and where necessary enforce these standards. Historically the key elements underpinning professions' self-regulating activities were the knowledge-base and associated educational curriculum, the requirements for becoming a member of the profession, and the code of ethics, conduct or practice. More recent pressures for greater accountability from professions, supported to some extent by a desire to create more diverse entry-routes, have led to increased concern with ensuring that new practitioners are suitably proficient at the point when they are signed off as fit to practise. This has led to many professions reinforcing the 'requirements for becoming a member' through explicit standards of competence or practice (Williams, Hanson, and Harrington 2013; Lester 2014a).

The interest of professions in competence and proficiency coupled with the now well-established extension of occupational standards to the upper levels of the occupational spectrum has created what appears to be a substantial overlap between the standards-related work of professional bodies and sector skills organisations. Although professional bodies are often represented on, or work with, SSCs, the use of the same standards by the two types of organisation is less common than might be expected. The reasons for this are potentially complex, although they stem partly from a difference between an occupational perspective on roles and competence and a professional one. The remainder of this paper draws on two main sources to explore this issue. The first is a study which I carried out in 2012 (Lester 2014a), involving examining standards and competence frameworks from 40 UK professions, supported by an earlier study of professional entry-routes and qualifying requirements (Lester 2008, 2009). The second is my work with four specific professions over the last 15 years as a developer or reviewer of professional standards and qualifying systems.

Occupations and occupational competence

An occupation, drawing on the Latin root *occupare* (to occupy), is an activity that takes up time: more specifically in the sense under discussion here, a (normally remunerative) role that occupies a person's working hours. An occupational perspective therefore has no special claims to make, in terms either of self-actualisation (as might a vocational standpoint to use that word in its correct sense) or of the need for commitment to any particular ethos (as might be the case from a professional viewpoint); it can simply be concerned with how the time is spent and therefore with factors such as quality and efficiency. This perspective is essentially utilitarian in nature, and is reflected in the way that the SSCs and their predecessors have gone about describing and creating standards for the work of occupations.

The two essential tools that have underpinned the UK occupational standards project are *occupational mapping*, essentially a research exercise to identify the nature and size of the occupation, the main roles within it and how they are organised, along with the main influences on its development; and *functional analysis*, an expert process to create standards by breaking the occupation down into successively more detailed work functions that contribute to achieving its purpose. These processes are described by Mitchell and Mansfield (1996), with more recent guidance provided by Carroll and Boutall (2010). Functional analysis is a develop-ment rather than a research technique, and although consultation is normally carried out as part of the process, it is a deductive method that depends for the quality of its results on the knowledge, currency and judgement of the expert group that carries it out. Three comments need to be made about functional analysis and occupational standards in the context of the discussion to follow. The first is that by using an approach that works downwards from the purpose of an occupation, functional anal-ysis creates a representation or map that attempts to define all the work that the occupation covers; typically this leads to a 'core-and-options' relationship between occupational standards and individual jobs, so that while some of the standards apply to all jobs, others will apply selectively. Second, because work is described by function, there is a tendency to differentiate between activities with different pur-poses even if the skills, knowledge and techniques needed to carry them out are essentially the same. Third, unsophisticated use of functional analysis tends not to distinguish the critical from the trivial, and many (particularly earlier) examples of occupational standards have been justly criticised for containing excessive and sometimes inane detail.

Doubts about the ability of this functional approach to provide a realistic reflec-tion of more than the most basic types of occupational competence have been voiced quite widely since the early 1990s. A particular critique has been that occupational standards are too static and closed to reflect the nature of complex work, where what is 'competent' both evolves and is subject to contextual factors (e.g. Elliott 1991; Burgoyne 1993; Grugulis 2000). There has also been widespread concern particu-larly from an educational perspective that in focusing on the outputs of competent activity, the competent person – and what it is that makes them competent – becomes lost (Gonczi, Hager, and Oliver 1990; Cheetham and Chivers 2005). The functional approach has nevertheless survived several reviews of occupational stan-dards and qualifications and two significant changes to the UK's vocational qualifi-cations frameworks, although recent reviews of different aspects of the vocational sector have criticised the standards once again as too prescriptive (Wolf 2011; Richard 2012; Whitehead 2013).

More positively, the approach taken in occupational standards has promoted an external, socially defined or activity-based version of competence based on being able to meet an explicit expectation (Eraut 1998). This contrasts with an internal view of competence (or competency) which focuses on the skills, knowledge and other attributes of individuals that are assumed to enable them to act competently. The external approach claims to be more holistic in that it represents the ability to use these attributes to achieve valued results, whereas from this perspective simply possessing skills, knowledge and attributes does not imply the ability to use them appropriately or effectively; to borrow a phrase, it may add up to no more than being 'a homunculus with a toolkit' (Holmes 1999, 89). Nevertheless both approaches have validity in relevant circumstances; internal models of competence are generally more useful for aiding development, while the external version is more geared to assessment and sign-off as fit to practise (Lester 2014a).

Professions and professional competence

In the English-speaking world the term 'profession' is sometimes used synony-mously with 'occupation' (as is the case in much of continental Europe), though its traditional usage is to refer to occupations associated with high levels of education and training and sometimes with well-developed systems of governance and self-regulation (e.g. Millerson 1964). However, the word's Latin root (*profiteri*, to declare publicly or make a vow) points to a more meaningful distinction in that being a member of a profession requires a formal commitment both to acquiring the relevant knowledge and skills and to the ethos and way of working of the profession, in a way that simply working in an occupation does not. While acknowledging the large body of literature on the nature of professions – useful discussions are provided by Abbott (1988), Freidson (2001) and Evetts (2003) among others – this more etymological notion is a useful one not least in that it focuses attention on *professionals* as active agents rather than *professions* as social constructs.

The way that professions conceptualise their core territories cannot be said to follow any one particular approach or perspective. Nevertheless, compared with the even mapping of activities that functional analysis aims to achieve, professions tend to be more oriented towards core capabilities that can be taken, applied and developed further by practitioners into areas centrally or more peripherally associated with the profession's work. This has at least partially grown out of the historic concern of professions with educational curricula and entry-routes (e.g. Schön 1983), rather than with definitions of work roles. Taking this approach, being (for instance) an architect is less concerned with a bounded description of what architects do than with acquiring the knowledge, skills, mindset and ethos of an architect; the practitioner may then do things other than what is normally understood as practising architecture, but remains an architect.

Professions' more recent interests in standards of competence and proficiency have brought them into contact with the occupationally oriented model, some features of which they have adopted. Their approaches to describing competence are however more varied than those that can be found in occupational standards, and recent trends are back towards a conception based on core capability rather than on the detailed mapping of functions (Lester 2014a). Initially it was fairly common for professions to use a largely internal approach to competence, i.e. to focus on the attributes needed by the practitioner. In a few cases this was simply concerned with the ability to apply the knowledge contained in the educational syllabus, but more sophisticated models also emerged drawing either on the instructional design tradition to identify in addition skills and personal attributes associated with the professional curriculum, or on the North American competency tradition (e.g. McClelland 1998) to identify attributes displayed by effective practitioners. Both the latter approaches lend themselves to a core capability perspective, the second particularly so, and they also support an orientation concerned with development rather than purely assessment. They do however have considerable disadvantages when used for assessment, particularly when the assessment is concerned with practice rather than learning (Lester 2014b). An increased focus on assessing practice, coupled with exposure over the last two decades to the occupational standards model, has tended to move professions away from internal approaches to competence and towards more external, activity-based conceptions; in my 2012 study (Lester 2014a), from a sample of 40 professions, 35 (88%) used a principally external approach to competence, and just under half of these described all aspects of professional capability in activity-based terms alone.

Despite the move to using external models of competence, it can be hypothesised that an underlying professional as opposed to occupational perspective remains and this influences the essential approach to conceptualising both the nature of the profession or occupation, as well as what is set out in the form of assessable standards. A few professions have simply adopted occupational standards or used functional analysis to create something similar, but these are now the exception. My 2012 study indicated first that professions devote significant attention to generic aspects of professionalism and professional activity, with things such as ethics, professional development, self-management and management of work, and communication or client relations accounting for on average over 40% of the content of professional competence frameworks. Second, what might be termed the functional areas of the profession tend to be described in terms of essential standards of practice rather than detailed work functions, with enough flexibility to apply across different contexts and allow for practices to evolve. Additionally, a majority of professions (65% in the study) favour generic frameworks, where the whole framework applies to all practitioners, as opposed to frameworks with different standards for different career pathways, specialisms or work contexts.

In some of the better-conceptualised professional frameworks there is a concern with what might be termed capability, in the sense used by Stephenson and Yorke (1998) and O'Reilly, Cunningham, and Lester (1999), as much as with competence and proficiency. Capability is arguably a less well-defined concept than competence, but an examination of the literature produced under the umbrella of the Higher Education for Capability movement (of which the above are prime examples) indicates that while, like competence, it is concerned with the ability to do, it also has a sense of being able to become (more) able to do, i.e. it also has a predictive element that goes beyond that present in the idea of competence. An (occupationally) competent practitioner should be able to act proficiently in a range of situations associated with the work of the occupation, but a capable practitioner can also be expected to develop competence as unforeseen contexts and new ways of working emerge. Frameworks influenced by a capability perspective tend to have as a core element a strong concern with the profession's ethics and ethos; they focus, in a carefully crafted way, on essential and durable standards of practice; and they use centre-outwards rather than bounded-occupation conceptions of the profession (Lester 2014b).

A further feature that is at least implicit in many professions' conceptualisations is that competence is seen as a scale rather than a fixed point. The occupational orthodoxy is that standards are set at a particular level – or multiple standards are created representing different levels of job – within which there is a single threshold separating competent performance from that which is not yet competent. This conception suggests a finite or closed notion of competence; although it is neutral as to whether updating is required to maintain currency, as a model it provides no recognition of development to higher levels of proficiency, and the unwritten assumption is that progression involves becoming competent in additional functions. Professions on the other hand tend to have a conception of practitioners developing their proficiency progressively, both up to and (critically) beyond the point at which they can be considered fully qualified or licensed to practise. This notion is reflected, if imperfectly, in the Dreyfus skills acquisition or 'novice-to-expert' model (Dreyfus and Dreyfus 1986) which is used explicitly by some professions as a development and assessment tool.

Professional standards in practice

The following short case-studies, drawn from four professions where I have been involved in developing or reviewing standards, are presented as a range of instances to illustrate how different professions have gone about defining their territory and setting out standards for practice. These are offered as examples rather than exemplars, illustrating how professional bodies adopt different approaches to articulating their perspectives on competence.

Conservation of cultural heritage

The activity of conserving and restoring items of material heritage has evolved gradually as a profession. University courses appeared in the 1930s, professional associations in the 1950s, a formally qualified designation was introduced in 1999, and the Institute of Conservation (Icon) was formed five years later. Professional standards were initially developed rather hurriedly and on a small budget to support assessment for qualified status; these comprised a functional section, drawing on (and condensing substantially) a set of pre-existing occupational standards (conservation was, after management, the first occupational area to develop standards at the old Level 5), and a section on judgement and ethics that was heavily influenced by a European development project, FULCO (Foley and Scholten 1998). The Dreyfus model was used explicitly as an aid to development and assessment. The original functional standards were quickly criticised for, effectively, being too occupational in style and restricting qualified status to too narrow a group of practitioners; they were essentially written for two specific work roles and proved divisive within the profession. An initial review involving expert groups enabled some tidying-up of the standards to make them more generic and easier to use, while a second review drew on research and consultation into what practitioners actually did as well as trials with groups previously excluded from coverage. The result was a move away from this functional approach, enabling a single set of professional standards to encompass a wide range of roles that included hands-on conservation treatment, environmental and other preventive measures, collections care management, advisory work, and (in terms of conservation expertise and competence) conservation teaching. The judgement and ethics standards were at the same time condensed, but presented and applied as central to all the other standards. The current standards document consists of 12 pages of text, including notes to aid assessment (see Icon 2007).

Despite the linkage between the occupational and professional standards, in some respects the approach to describing competence taken in conservation epitomises the difference between an occupational and a professional model. The standards start from the core of the profession – the ethos and ethics, the essential decision-making processes involved in conserving heritage – and are written in a way that both avoids the detail of specific roles and provides room for practice to evolve, while making clear the standard that is needed. This ensures that they can apply across specialisms and, more critically, across different roles. Perhaps interestingly they have been used to inform the development of revised occupational standards and transfer some of the breadth of the professional approach back into them.

Landscape architecture

Landscape architecture is a well-established profession with an institute formed in 1929 and a Royal Charter since 1997. Entry is at postgraduate level, and all would-be practitioners are required to undergo a period (normally in the region of two years) of supervised practice and training which is assessed formatively in the work-place and summatively through a presentation and oral examination. Until recently, this assessment was based on what was effectively a knowledge-based syllabus. The Landscape Institute developed a set of professional standards ('elements of practice') in 2010–11 (Landscape Institute 2012), largely following the conservation model in style and level of detail. These were designed in principle to apply across the profession's five current specialisms, although early testing suggested that not all areas of the standards worked equally well for each. As with the later conservation standards, they were set at the level of a proficient, experienced practitioner and designed to encompass a broad range of roles as well as current and potential future specialisms. A key difference is that the standards are not used directly for assessment, but represent a guide to proficient practice; a subset of the main standards, scaled back to competent or advanced beginner level, has been produced for assessment after the training period, and it is also intended to use the standards to inform course approval processes.

Similar comments apply to the landscape architecture standards as to those in conservation, except that there were no suitable occupational standards available to aid development. Conservation uses its standards directly for assessment (generally assuming around five years' or more experience on the part of candidates), with a few additional notes of explanation to guide assessors and aid candidates. To date the promotion of the conservation standards for other purposes, such as acting as a general standard of practice or informing clients of what can be expected from conservators, has been limited despite the fact that they are eminently suitable for doing this. Landscape architecture on the other hand views the standards more as a blueprint that can be used to convey a general standard of practice to members, clients and the public, as well as to develop the more specific applications referred to above.

Vocational rehabilitation

Vocational rehabilitation (VR) is concerned with the return to work of people with disabilities and long-term illnesses. Many practitioners will already have qualified in areas such as physiotherapy, occupational therapy, careers guidance or vocational education, and as yet there is no widely accepted qualified status in VR. The VR Association published a set of professional standards in 2007, amounting to 128 pages and reading as an extended code of practice; this was developed roughly in parallel with a British Standard for service providers. While the professional standards document attracted criticism for being excessively detailed, not particularly well-structured and in some places too restrictive, it was also seen as capturing much of the researched and practical wisdom about effective VR practice. The document was revised in 2012–13 to a set of statements contained in 16 pages (Vocational Rehabilitation Association 2013) that expressed the ethos and ethics of VR as well as providing functional standards for core activities. These are designed to apply to a broad range of VR contexts, and include a mixture of highly general sections and those that relate to specific functions and are more occupational in character. At present the standards are used for guidance and self-assessment, and while they have been through a consultation process they have not been subjected to detailed testing to determine how well they apply to the work that individual VR practitioners actually do.

The VR standards aim, like those for conservation and landscape architecture, to apply to all practitioners. The standards are however more specific in the way that they describe work processes, reflecting their origins as a code of practice; ignoring the presentational style, the function-specific sections of the standards take a more occupational perspective than the previous two examples. Detailed testing of the standards may indicate that they need to be applied via a core-and-options approach, albeit with the majority of the standards forming the core.

Personnel and development

The personnel and development community is represented by the Chartered Institute of Personnel and Development (CIPD), established in 1994 from a merger of pre-existing bodies dating back to 1913; its charter was granted in 2000. Various routes are available to chartered membership, including a postgraduate course followed by relevant experience, progression from lower grades of membership, and direct assessment for experienced practitioners. The CIPD initially used what was effectively a syllabus in place of professional standards, choosing not to adopt existing occupational standards due to concerns about their relevance, currency and (lack of) depth. These 'standards' were replaced in 2008–09 by a 'profession map' based on 10 functional areas, each described at four levels equating broadly to job roles between assistant and director level and expressed in terms of key activities and underpinning knowledge. Each functional area is also referenced to eight behavioural areas, again expressed at four levels. The CIPD profession map (CIPD 2012) has proved considerably more successful and versatile than the earlier syllabus-based standards. However, it has also attracted a certain amount of criticism in being too limited in terms of the roles it covers, these being geared to the human resources function in large organisations and less easily applicable to (for instance) sole personnel practitioners in small firms or external consultants and service providers. Some minor amendments have been made to the map since its inception, but it retains the same basic structure and focus.

The CIPD profession map differs from the preceding examples in several respects. First, it contains standards at different levels, although this is no different from areas such as engineering where different grades of qualified membership are defined (Icon, somewhat similarly, uses what is effectively a subset of its standards for a qualification at technician level). Second, the function-based standards are organised by role (e.g. employee relations, learning and development, organisation development) with what is effectively a small common core, in contrast with the more generic approach of the examples described above. Third, the map includes separate specifications for knowledge – generally expressed as context-specific factual knowledge – which is normally left as implicit in most professional standards frameworks. Finally, the presence of behavioural competencies is now uncommon in professional or occupational standards, though shared with the occupational standards for management; both this and the knowledge content partly reflect that the map is intended to be a development (including self-development) tool as much as a framework for assessment. Overall this suggests that the CIPD map reflects at least partly an occupational standpoint, although it provides a deeper and more capability-oriented perspective than the corresponding occupational standards (see Skills CFA 2012).

Conclusion: a professional perspective on work competence

The examples above and the research study both suggest that there is no single recipe for professional competence standards parallel to that used in UK occupational standards, but they do concur with the notion of a distinctive professional perspective on competence. Translating this into a set of principles for a competence framework suggests the following:

- First, the work of the profession is normally covered by a single universal set of standards: there is not normally a core-and-options structure relating to different functions, but standards are set in a way that allows for them to be interpreted into different contexts and for practices to evolve. The framework generally conceptualises the profession in terms of a set of ethics, principles and key standards, emphasising activities and requirements that apply across the profession's work rather than attempting to map detailed functions and tasks.
- Second, the standards are designed to provide a measure of confidence in practitioners' ability not only to act competently in specific situations, but to work effectively – currently and into the future – within the profession. There is generally an assumption that development will continue beyond the threshold or licence-to-practise level, even if this is not made explicit through something like the Dreyfus novice-to-expert model. Assessments using the standards will look for contextual competence, but they will treat it as providing an example of wider professional capability, and typically they will also want to see more holistic evidence of the ability to understand situations in depth and make sound professional judgements.
- Finally, accreditation of an individual according to a professional model is endorsement as a member of the profession, not to do a specific job; the scope of the individual's practice becomes a matter of ethics (not practising or 'holding out' to practise unsupervised in areas where competence and expertise are lacking) and if necessary disciplinary measures, rather than (normally) needing reference to additional standards or assessments.

These principles represent an archetypal or ideal model that reflects the notion of a profession based on value-commitment as opposed to an occupation concerned more purely with role performance. Of the four examples discussed in detail, this model is most evident in conservation and landscape architecture. Conservation follows the principles almost in their entirety, despite covering a large number of technical specialisms as well as accommodating a broad range of work roles; landscape architecture is currently in transition from an older model where entrants qualified in one of three divisions, to one where the number of specialisms is increasing and the boundaries between them are blurring, focusing attention on the profession as a whole rather than on discrete divisions. In vocational rehabilitation the view has prevailed that more detailed attention is needed to the key occupational role of the profession, partly because this is seen as critical for raising standards and effectiveness; it may also stem, in an area that is less mature as a profession than the two previous examples, from a concern to ensure that the standards explicitly communicate good practice. In personnel and development the CIPD's 'map' reflects the diverse roles and specialisms within the human resources function, for which it provides a reasonably sophisticated and practical structure. On the other hand, it gives far less of a sense of a coherent profession than the other three sets of standards. While parallel if different solutions have been adopted in a few other diverse professions (surveying is a notable example), there may also be a question as to whether the CIPD's constituency can be conceptualised as a single profession.

In practice, the approach taken by any profession to describing work competence will need to reflect its particular make-up, operating context and expectations. My 2012 study found a large variation in the quality of competence frameworks used by professions, but as illustrated here, there is substantial variation in approach even among well-researched and thought-out frameworks. In reality, 'professions' are not all of the same type, nor are 'occupations'; even using the simple etymological definitions given earlier in this paper, any given area of work, viewed from any of several perspectives, is likely to have a mix of professional and occupational characteristics. This suggests that the kind of competence model that is appropriate will range from the archetypally professional to the pragmatically occupational, with various mixed models in between. This has implications for professions, in that while there are some guiding principles and potential exemplars there is no single methodology for developing professional standards. A similar caveat must also apply to occupational standards, as many occupations have some of the characteristics of professions and they may not be best served by conceptions of competence that are, in the terms used here, narrowly occupational.

References

Abbott, A. 1988. *The System of Professions*. Chicago, IL: University of Chicago Press.
Burgoyne, J. 1993. "The Competence Movement: Issues, Stakeholders and Prospects." *Personnel Review* 22 (6): 6–13.
Carroll, G., and T. Boutall. 2010. *Guide to Developing National Occupational Standards*. Wath-upon-Dearne: UK Commission for Employment and Skills. Accessed October 31, 2013. http://www.ukces.org.uk/assets/ukces/docs/supporting-docs/nos/guide-to-developing-nos.pdf
Chartered Institute of Personnel and Development (CIPD). 2012. *HR Profession Map*. London: CIPD. Accessed December 31, 2013. https://www.cipd.co.uk/cipd-hr-profession/profession-map/profession-map-download.aspx
Cheetham, G., and G. Chivers. 2005. *Professions, Competence and Informal Learning*. Cheltenham: Edward Elgar.
Dreyfus, H. L., and S. E. Dreyfus. 1986. *Mind over Machine: The Power of Human Intuition and Expertise in the Era of the Computer*. Oxford: Blackwell.

Elliott, J. 1991. *Action Research for Educational Change*. Buckingham: Open University Press.

Eraut, M. 1998. "Concepts of Competence." *Journal of Interprofessional Care* 12 (2): 127–139.

Evetts, J. 2003. "The Sociological Analysis of Professionalism: Occupational Change in the Modern World." *International Sociology* 18 (2): 395–415.

Foley, K., and S. Scholten. 1998. *FULCO: A Framework of Competence for Conservator-Restorers in Europe*. Amsterdam: Instituut Collectie Nederland.

Freidson, E. 2001. *Professionalism: The Third Logic*. Cambridge: Polity.

Gonczi, A., P. Hager, and L. Oliver. 1990. *Establishing Competency-based Standards in the Professions*. Canberra: Australian Government Publishing Service.

Grugulis, I. 2000. "The Management NVQ: A Critique of the Myth of Relevance." *Journal of Vocational Education and Training* 52 (1): 79–99.

Holmes, L. 1999. "Competence and Capability: From 'Confidence Trick' to the Construction of Graduate Identity." In *Developing the Capable Practitioner*, edited by D. O'Reilly, L. Cunningham, and S. Lester, 83–98. London: Routledge.

Icon (Institute of Conservation). 2007. *Revised Professional Standards for Conservation*. London: Icon. Accessed October 31, 2013. http://www.sld.demon.co.uk/iconstds.doc

Landscape Institute. 2012. *Landscape Architecture: Elements and Areas of Practice*. London: Landscape Institute. Accessed October 31, 2013. http://www.landscapeinstitute.org/PDF/Contribute/A4_Elements_and_areas_of_practice_education_framework_Board_final_2012.pdf

Lester, S. 2008. *Routes and Requirements for Becoming Professionally Qualified*. Bristol: Professional Associations Research Network.

Lester, S. 2009. "Routes to Qualified Status: Practices and Trends among UK Professional Bodies." *Studies in Higher Education* 34 (2): 223–236.

Lester, S. 2014a. "Professional Competence Standards and Frameworks in the UK." *Assessment and Evaluation in Higher Education* 39 (1): 38–52.

Lester, S. 2014b. "Professional Standards, Competence and Capability." *Higher Education, Skills and Work-based Learning* 4 (1): 31–43.

McClelland, D. C. 1998. "Identifying Competencies with Behavioral-event Interviews." *Psychological Science* 9 (5): 331–339.

Millerson, G. 1964. *The Qualifying Associations: A Study in Professionalization*. London: Routledge and Kegan Paul.

Mitchell, L., and B. Mansfield. 1996. *Towards a Competent Workforce*. Aldershot: Gower.

O'Reilly, D., L. Cunningham, and S. Lester, eds. 1999. *Developing the Capable Practitioner*. London: Routledge.

Richard, D. 2012. *The Richard Review of Apprenticeships*. London: School for Startups.

Schön, D. A. 1983. *The Reflective Practitioner: How Professionals Think in Action*. New York: Jossey-Bass.

Skills CFA. 2012. *Human Resources National Occupational Standards*. London: Skills CFA. Accessed October 31, 2013. http://www.skillscfa.org/images/pdfs/National%20Occupational%20Standards/Human%20Resources%20and%20Recruitment/2011/Human%20Resources.pdf

Stephenson, J., and M. Yorke, eds. 1998. *Capability and Quality in Higher Education*. London: Kogan Page.

Vocational Rehabilitation Association (VRA). 2013. *Standards of Practice and Code of Ethics for Vocational Rehabilitation Practitioners*. Doncaster: VRA. Accessed October 31, 2013. http://www.vra-uk.org/civicrm/contribute/transact?reset=1&id=10

Whitehead, N. (Chair). 2013. *Review of Adult Vocational Qualifications in England*. Wath-upon-Dearne: UK Commission for Employment and Skills.

Williams, C., W. Hanson, and A. Harrington. 2013. *Framing Professional Competence: Lessons for Professional Bodies on Creating, Using and Reviewing Competency Frameworks*. Bristol: Professional Associations Research Network.

Wolf, A. 2011. *Review of Vocational Education – The Wolf Report*. London: Department for Education and Department for Business and Skills. Accessed October 31, 2013. https://www.gov.uk/government/publications/review-of-vocational-education-the-wolf-report

Professionalism in vocational education: international perspectives

Liz Atkins ⓘ and Jonathan Tummons ⓘ

ABSTRACT

This paper explores notions of professionalism amongst vocational teachers in the United Kingdom and Australia, through an analysis of voluntarism/regulatory frameworks and professional body frameworks. In terms of empirical evidence, the paper reports on data drawn from a documentary analysis of government policy documents, standards for the education of teachers, and regulatory frameworks in both countries. It is located within a broad range of literature exploring contemporary concepts of professionalism amongst vocational teachers. Documentary analysis implies that whilst there is an expectation and assumption that vocational teachers are, and should be, professional, this is not necessarily translated through initial teacher training requirements, some of which fail to address concepts of professionalism at all. Further, it offers evidence to suggest that where notions of professionalism are addressed, the concept is described in largely reductive and utilitarian terms, and that this is the case in both countries. The paper considers the implications of this for teachers, students, and wider practice within the sector, arguing that meaningful understandings of the notion of professional, which are effectively applied in practice, are fundamental to broader understandings of key issues in further education, such as those associated with in/equalities and in/exclusion in education contexts. The paper concludes that such understandings are unlikely to be drawn from utilitarian, Competency Based Training (CBT) based teacher-training programmes.

Exploring discourses of professionalism

Professionalism can be understood as a fluid concept with a range of different meanings and interpretations, changing over time and according to context. Eraut (1994) for example, describes professionalism as an ideology characterised by specialist knowledge, autonomy and service, whilst Winch (2014) defines professionalism through an exploration of the relationship of agency to professional capacity. Other interpretations refer to knowledge, power, and relationships with society (see Evetts 2013, for an extended discussion).

Much of the literature uses the so-called elite professions of law and medicine as exemplars, and draws on conceptions of 'professional' which are juxtaposed with historical constructions of 'vocational': an occupational role such as teaching or nursing, defined in terms of calling or service. The focus on law and medicine can be dated back to landmark studies in professionalism such as that of Millerson (1964), who explored these two professions through the construction of a five-part framework for defining a profession as any occupation which required use of skills based on theoretical knowledge; receipt of education or training in those skills; accredited and examined certificates to practice; a code of professional conduct; and a commitment to the 'public good'. It is important to note that in an earlier study of further education (FE) professionalism in England, Clow (2005) argued that, following a strict application of the Millerson model of professionalism, teaching in FE could not be classed as a profession.

In the context of further education, the meanings and interpretations most commonly used fall within two opposing paradigms, which are framed within different types of discourse (Gee 1996; Lemke 1995). These discourses may be understood in one of three ways: as being positioned within a managerialist paradigm, an emancipatory paradigm, or a utilitarian paradigm (Avis 2007; Kennedy 2007; Tummons 2014a). Here, we define the managerialist paradigm of professionalism as emphasising audit and performativity through the application of 'professional' standards (Shore and Wright 2000). According to this discourse, professional standards, and any related regulatory frameworks such as inspection regimes or quality assurance processes, are positioned as forms of social control imposed upon teachers, masked behind a discourse of 'improving standards' which serves instead to control teachers' labour and impose a model of professionalism from above or outside the profession itself. In contrast to this, an emancipatory model of professionalism is positioned as one in which professional standards and associated regulatory frameworks come under the purview of the members of the profession, which espouses more democratic, emancipatory notions of professionalism (Evetts 2013; Gleeson, Davies, and Wheeler 2005; Petrie 2015, p.6). Distinct from both of these is the utilitarian paradigm. This discourse of professionalism can be understood as being a product of new managerialism (Randle and Brady, 1997a, 1997b; Shain and Gleeson 1999), resting on a simultaneous de-skilling and intensification of labour amongst the FE teaching workforce. Within this discourse, professionalism is positioned entirely in terms of acceptance of and adherence to working practices that position the FE teacher as a technician, ignoring the importance or value of subject expertise and instead focusing on generic teaching skills.

It is important to note that these discourses do not necessarily exist in isolation or apart from each other. By this we mean to stress that it is possible to find traces of all three of these discourses at work at the same time, during the last 20 years (the timespan for the current investigation). It is worth noting that before the UK coalition government's deregulation of the FE sector in 2010, the prevailing professionalisation agenda was narrow, instrumental and controlling (for example, by requiring teachers to join the now-defunct Institute for Learning), but at the same time offered meaningful opportunities for funded professional training such as PGCE/Cert Ed for all full-time FE teachers, which offered the opportunity to debate issues around professionalism beyond the narrow interpretations imposed by the sector and reflected in both the Further Education National Training Organisation (FENTO) and Lifelong Learning UK (LLUK) professional standards. The return to voluntary professional qualifications in the FE sector was positioned by the coalition government within a discourse of flexibility and responsiveness to employers: simply put, it was argued that college principals would know better than government departments what their workforces required in terms of professional training and development. And yet standards and regulation remained in place: indeed, a new set of standards – the Education and Training Foundation (ETF) standards – was published. But what was now lacking was the funding for teachers to undertake advanced forms of training (such as that offered in universities) and Continuing Professional Development (CPD) beyond that deemed appropriate by their employing institution.

Contrasting national systems: the UK and Australia

For the purpose of this discussion, we draw on the various iterations of UK professional standards for FE practitioners, the requirements of a range of qualifications and the policy and regulatory frameworks and contexts in which they sit. We refer to the UK where frameworks relate to all countries in the union, and England where policy or frameworks are specific to that country. We contrast these with the Australian nationally mandated Certificate IV in Training and Assessment (Cert IV TAE), federal and state regulatory frameworks and the draft standards for further education and training (FET) teachers proposed by the Queensland College of Teachers. Across all documents, we utilise the nomenclature of those documents: this means that the terms vocational education, VET, and FE are used interchangeably. The first set of professional standards for further education teachers in the UK was published in 1999 after a consultation period of several years, followed two years later by statutory reform that made the acquisition of appropriate initial teaching qualifications based on the standards compulsory for new teachers in the sector (Nasta 2007). The standards were published by FENTO: one of a larger number of national training organisations (NTOs) introduced by the UK Conservative government of 1979–1997 to specify and implement relevant education and training programmes for the sector in question. The FENTO standards were criticised by some university-based researchers for being overly instrumental, technicist, and undervaluing wider professional development (Elliott 2000). They were also criticised by Ofsted, in their 2003 report *The Initial Training of Further Education Teachers* (HMI 1762: Ofsted 2003). According to this report, teacher education in the sector was seen as being too variable and too inconsistent despite the introduction of new standards and new qualifications and as lacking subject-specialist pedagogy (Lucas 2004).

In the following year, the then Department for Education and Skills (2004) published a new working paper, *Equipping Our Teachers for the Future*, which promised reform of LLS teacher education as part of a wider change in workforce education and training. NTOs were gradually replaced by new organisations – Sector Skills Councils (SSCs) – and FENTO was subsequently replaced by LLUK, who published a new set of standards in 2006, after another period of consultation. These standards were accompanied by a further element: a new process of professional formation that required teachers in the LLS sector to achieve a new professional status – Qualified Teacher, Learning and Skills (QTLS) – following a compulsory period of continuing professional development (CPD). Criticism remained: from university researchers, who argued that the new standards were still mechanistic, overly prescriptive and narrowed the content of teacher education curricula (Lucas, Nasta, and Rogers 2012), and from policymakers who allowed the standards to ossify, first by abolishing LLUK, and second by removing financial support from the Institute for Learning (the professional body for LLS teachers that, amongst other things, was responsible for auditing teachers' CPD and QTLS endorsement) which ceased operations at the end of 2014. The QTLS process of professional formation has survived, but the management of the process has been passed from the IFL (ostensibly a member-led organisation) to the Education and Training Foundation (very much an employer-led organisation).

The impact of this has been that whilst some universities have closed their provision, others still continue to offer higher education teaching qualifications at a number of levels – Certificate in Education (Cert. Ed. level 5), sometimes Professional Graduate Certificate in Education (ProfGCE, level 6) or Post Graduate Certificate in Education (PGCE, level 7). Awarding bodies have developed qualifications based on the most recent standards, which retain the nomenclature of those under the 2007 standards. The Diploma in Teaching in the Lifelong Learning Sector (popularly known as D[e]TLLS), is a competency based credential of seven core and four optional units, offered at level 5. Whilst one of these is 'continuing personal and professional development', the competencies do not engage with understandings of what it means to be a professional. There are a range of other credentials offered, which are shorter/lower in level. Of these, the Preparing to Teach in Lifelong Learning (PTLLS) level 4 credential bears the closest similarity to the Australian Cert IV. Notions of professionalism are absent from the competencies forming this credential, as they are from the more extended Level 4 Certificate in Teaching in the Lifelong Learning Sector, and, indeed, the Cert IV itself.

The Australian vocational education and training system, formed by a combination of technical and further education colleges (TAFEs) and registered training organisations (RTOs), broadly equivalent to UK private training providers, has significant similarities to the English and Welsh systems, although there is less broad vocational education and a higher proportion of training that takes place in the work place. Regulatory frameworks also have striking similarities to those in the UK, but are complicated by the fact that some aspects of the sector (regulatory frameworks for providers for example) are within the remit of national government, whilst funding and related aspects of policy are the responsibility of the autonomous state governments. This can lead to variations between states even where a policy is nationally implemented. For example, the Diploma in Vocational Education and Training (VET) teaching, an optional qualification which also consists of centrally defined standards and achievement of which moves the holder to an identified upper point on the national pay scales, requires students to undertake 200 hours classroom practice in Victoria but in neighbouring New South Wales, no classroom practice is necessary.

As in the UK, there is no financial incentive for teachers in Australia who work in the VET sector to undertake study at degree or master's level. This is despite the fact that, originally, there was a consensus that VET teachers should hold teaching qualifications with graduate status, equivalent to those held by school teachers – an equivalence echoed in the short-lived LLUK framework that sought to create equivalence between school teachers and college lecturers through the Qualified Teacher, Learning and Skills (QTLS) status which would be akin to QTS for school teachers. Instead, the 1990s saw a move in Australia from a higher level of mandated qualification to a minimalist one (Guthrie 2010). Guthrie proposes a range of reasons for this, key amongst which are the cost of higher education programmes to the funders, casualization of the VET workforce, concomitant with limited access to training and CPD, and a greater focus on the workplace, rather than the classroom, as a site of learning – all issues which are familiar to those involved with the UK system.

Consequent to this deregulation, the Cert IV became the only nationally mandated credential required for teachers working in the VET sector in Australia. The qualification is offered by Universities, TAFEs and RTOs, and is generally acknowledged as being of variable quality. It is a 30-hour programme broadly similar in size, content and level to the now defunct PTLLS award in the UK, but significant in its lack of coverage of assessment within the syllabus, something which has led to a number of arguments within and beyond the sector that assessment practices are weak and inconsistent. The inadequacy of the Certificate IV as a minimum credential is also acknowledged in the draft version of the *Professional Standards for Vocational Education and Training Practitioners (PSVETP)* (Queensland College of Teachers, 2015, 2), originally planned for implementation in Queensland in 2016, in part as a response to perceived weaknesses in the Certificate IV. Notwithstanding concerns over the syllabus, the Certificate IV still has advocates. For example, Clayton (2009) cites National Assessors and Workplace Trainers (NAWT) (2001), who argued that the Certificate IV was critical to the VET sector in two ways: first, in providing standards for trainers and assessors to adhere to; and second, in providing structural support for the quality assurance arrangements of RTOs.

Models of professionalism across national contexts

In comparison to a relatively lively, as well as long-standing, body of literature discussing professionalism in vocational education and training in England and Wales, there is a paucity of literature exploring how professionalism is understood in the context of VET teaching in Australia. Nonetheless, some authors (e.g. see Robertson 2008), have raised concerns that the Certificate IV TAE requirements are not consistent with the development of 'expert' and 'professional' teachers, but only with those for novice or beginning teachers. That is to say, the Certificate IV requirements are seen as being appropriate only at entry to the profession, a critique that resonates with similar earlier criticisms of the English FENTO standards and the qualifications that were mapped onto these (Lucas 2004). However, whereas subsequent series of professional standards in the UK have made sincere, if contested, attempts to establish consensual models of professionalism within the sector, in Australia there has been a failure to define professionalism, except insofar as it is conflated with notions of the 'expert' teacher, and the literature tends to focus on the lack of content within the Cert IV. For example, Simons, Harris, and Smith (2006) criticised the absence of any reference to learning theory, as well as the uncritical application of concepts such as learning styles, whilst Robertson (2008) argued that (in a previous incarnation) the Certificate IV programme had no evidence of critique or conceptual foundations, also noting a complete absence of critique of CBT: indeed, he goes further, arguing that the Cert IV was mandated as the minimum qualification for VET teachers in Australia as part of an attempt to de-professionalise teachers and create technicist trainers.

More recently, work by Williams (2010) provides a snapshot of different debates around actions which might improve VET teacher education. As with some of the debates discussed earlier in this paper, she acknowledges the absence of knowledge in the Cert. IV, and goes on to consider changes to teacher education that could improve the professional knowledge base. However, notions of professionalism are not interrogated, but the concept of being a 'professional' teacher is conflated with the acquisition of particular teaching qualifications. Similarly, Smith, Hodge, and Yasukawa (2015: 421) identify the Australian Qualifications Framework (AQF) outcomes for different levels of training, in which level 4 is identified as equating to 'skilled work' but 'level 7 to 'professional work', again implying a qualification-led, instrumental definition of professionalism. Participants in their study reported that their teacher education programmes were making a very positive contribution to personal and professional development. However, this raises questions about how the notion of professional development is being constructed by the participants, and by those who are preparing them for entry into teaching. Weaknesses in the preparation of teachers to work in the Australian VET sector have also been acknowledged by Moodie and Wheelahan (2012), who have questioned understandings of subject-appropriate pedagogies in different occupational fields. Like Williams they consider possible changes to VET teacher preparation, and argue that the development of a model for improvement would require the support of institutions and processes which should include a professional association, standards for teaching, and accreditation of teaching qualifications. Such processes, if adopted in Australia, would be broadly comparable to those which have taken place in England as part of ongoing attempts to 're-professionalise' the sector by governments with a diversity of ideological approaches. Notably, the development of the Queensland standards implies that these processes are beginning, albeit on a state, rather than national scale.

Professionalism, curriculum and professional standards

It is quite common for professional bodies to endorse specific qualifications that are designed to provide students with the required practical and/or theoretical competence, knowledge and experience, at a threshold level, to allow them entry to the profession in question. Through aligning professional curricula with professional standards, the qualifications in question can then be benchmarked in terms of delivery, performance and assessment, all in such a way as to meet the requirements of the relevant professional body (Katz 2000; Taylor 1997). It follows, then, that if a qualification such as a Certificate in Education or a Diploma in Teaching and Learning in the Lifelong Learning Sector has been endorsed by one of the three professional bodies that have since 1999 had purview of the sector (FENTO, LLUK or ETF), and then also been mapped onto the appropriate professional framework or set of standards, aspects of those standards would be found embedded in the curriculum being followed. These have been explored in detail elsewhere (Tummons 2014a, 2014b). At the same time, we might expect similar processes to take place within equivalent curricula in Australia, a theme to which we now turn.

The TAE programme in Australia consists of 10 units – seven core and three optional – all described and assessed within the context of a CBT framework that includes performance criteria, range statements and knowledge criteria. Across all seven core units there is just one single reference to professionalism, in a single criterion which requires the candidate to be able to

> use appropriate communication and interpersonal skills to develop *a professional relationship* with the candidate that reflects sensitivity to individual differences and enables two-way feedback, (TAEASS402B; emphasis added)

However, the criterion is not underpinned by a requirement to understand concepts of professionalism at any level. Without such foundations, therefore, how can the VET practitioner be conceptualised as a professional? What meanings can legitimately be applied to the term 'professional relationship'? The inclusion of even this minor reference to a 'professional relationship' implies an assumption that teachers will be able to conceptualise the nature of a 'professional relationship' and enact that in their day-to-day working lives. However, any reference to these conceptual foundations is absent from the TAE requirements which fail to address even the most instrumental analyses of what it means to be professional.

In stark contrast to the TAE requirements, the newly published Queensland College of Teachers (QCT) standards (2015) are structured around three domains of *professional knowledge, professional practice* and *professional learning and engagement*, suggesting that those responsible for the development of the standards have concerns about the way in which VET teachers enact their role, and the extent to which this might be described as professional. Similarly, the revised frameworks for training providers introduced as part of the ongoing Australian Federal VET Reform policy make only passing reference to the term professional, and then in the context of 'professional development', which is defined as maintaining the 'knowledge and practice of vocational training, learning and assessment' (Commonwealth of Australia 2015; para 1.16). However, whilst the QCT draft standards mention 'professionalism' with considerable frequency, it is, perhaps unsurprisingly, not explicitly defined. Moreover, despite the frequency with which the word is reiterated, there is no change to the meaning of the text if Kennedy's (2007) test of removing the word 'professional' is applied. For example, Domain 3, *Professional* Learning and Engagement includes standard 6 'Engage in *Professional* Learning in your vocational area and in adult education theories and practices', the criteria for which are:

6.1 participate in ongoing professional learning to maintain and update subject area and/or vocational knowledge and skills;

6.2 undertake ongoing professional learning in contemporary principles and practices of teaching/training, learning and assessment; and

6.3 engage in professional dialogue as part of a process of personal continuous improvement and professional growth.

(Queensland College of Teachers (QCT) 2015, p.4; our emphasis)

Removal of the word professional makes no difference to what is expected of those teachers to whom the standards apply. This would seem to suggest that utilitarian, rather than emancipatory understandings and discourses of professionalism are embedded within these standards even though they imply a degree of agency and autonomy which is considerably broader than that conferred by the Cert IV. Beyond the standards themselves, the QCT provides a glossary of terms (ibid, p. 5), where, for example, the 'domains of teaching' are described as 'professional knowledge, professional practice and professional engagement'. In this context, the word *pedagogic* might be more descriptive of what teaching actually involves.

The construction of the 'professional' is similarly problematic within both the current UK standards (Education and Training Foundation 2014) as well as the previous two iterations (FENTO 1999; LLUK 2007). That is to say, the ways in which what it means to be a 'professional' teacher in further education are constructed in terms of occupational performativity rather than an ethic or philosophy of professionalism. Arguably, it is hardly surprising that any rich or nuanced understanding of professionalism is absent in a document consisting of just 346 words. More extensive guidance is provided in an accompanying document, *Initial Guidance For Users of the Professional Standards*. This document provides an extensive discussion of how the standards might be used in practice. Alongside a strong focus on professional learning and continuing professional development (which are, arguably, operating as tropes within the document as a whole) can be found references to professional knowledge, professional development, professional behaviour, professional conduct, and so forth. But none of these are clearly defined or pinned to an ethos or philosophy. The document posits itself as providing a series of guidelines that can be applied or enacted within individual organisations but fails to acknowledge the politics of such an implementation. Teachers in FE are encouraged to take responsibility for their own professional learning (whatever that might mean), but are not encouraged to take responsibility for the discursive constructions of professionalism within which they are enrolled as social actors (Gee 1996).

The guidance document presents itself as being 'research based' (Education and Training Foundation 2014: 5): a position that is to be welcomed alongside 2014 professional standard number 8, that asks practitioners to 'maintain and update your knowledge of educational research to develop evidence-based practice'. But how rigorous is this research? The research base for both the standards and for the guidance document is to be found in an earlier document, commissioned by the Education and Training Foundation, and conducted by RCU, a research and consultancy company (Fletcher et al. 2013). Within the standards, one of the constructs used is that of *dual professionalism*, an important as well as complex issue that has been the subject of serious academic research and critique (Gleeson, Davies, and Wheeler 2005; Orr and Simmons 2010; Plowright and Barr 2012). But there is no mention of any such research within the RCU document. This is a document which is based on 66 sources, but only two of these can be seen as being examples of serious and rigorous academic work and only one of these takes professionalism in further education as its subject, albeit written before the introduction of the *first* set of professional standards by FENTO (Robson 1998). For a mature profession that seeks to situate itself within a serious research-informed and evidence-led approach to pedagogy, surely a more critical and thorough exploration of dual professionalism is needed?

It is not necessary, however, for professional standards – either in Australia or in the UK – to provide an explicit definition of any or all of the terms or constructs that they draw upon: professional standards do lots of things, but they do not provide glossaries; nor are they expected to. But the dominant discourses (Gee 1996) within which they are located will construct 'professionalism' in particular ways. We suggest, therefore, that it is through the textual analysis of the standards that latent constructs of professionalism can be made visible.

QCT standard 1.1 is the only one of the proposed Queensland standards which explicitly requires theoretical knowledge, and then only in relation to the underpinning of 'effective practice' in teaching and assessment. In the UK, whilst professional standards 8 and 9 require practitioners to 'maintain and update your knowledge of educational research to develop evidence based practice' and 'apply theoretical understanding of effective practice in teaching, learning and assessment drawing on research and other evidence', these criteria too imply that theoretical underpinnings of teaching as practice are all that is necessary for teachers to understand, a position which may be argued to privilege 'knowing how' over 'knowing that' (Winch 2015; after Ryle 1949), as well as reflecting a failure to acknowledge the symbiotic relationship between the two types of knowledge.

Knowledge and professionalism

The lack of acknowledgement of a meaningful base of propositional knowledge for teachers (Shulman 1986; and see also Eraut 1994) across both national contexts at best marginalises, and at worst dismisses the foundational subjects which underpin the study of education: the history, philosophy, sociology and psychology of education – implying that somehow, they are of no particular relevance to the workshop or classroom as these are currently positioned by policymakers, reflecting the use of an instrumental CBT approach to teacher education. Teacher education thus becomes a form of 'pseudo-apprenticeship' which de-professionalises the intending teacher as they do not require mastery of inbuilt theory (Broudy 1972), in stark contrast to the concept of professional education as being based around the provision of a threshold body of knowledge as well as competence and ethical practice, appropriate for new entrants to the profession in question (Taylor 1997).

In the context of the body of knowledge required for new entrants to teaching in the FE sector in both England and Australia, a number of observations might be made in relation to both the content of the minimum credentials as well as the construction of the curriculum itself, and the implications this has for the way in which FE teachers construct notions of professionalism. In terms of the competency-based approach, a number of criticisms might be made. First, as Bathmaker (2013, p. 91) has argued, a key issue in debates about knowledge in vocational education is the tension between conceptualisations of knowledge and conceptualisations of skill. This observation is also clearly relatable to (vocationally orientated and competency-based) teacher training for the sector. Further, as Bathmaker also argues, in the context of the FE sector, conceptions of skill are fluid, but currently understood in terms of (neo-liberal) discourses around attitudes and dispositions, as well as employability.

A number of authors have explored the nature of knowledge, and have found it to be incompatible with the instrumental conceptualisations of skill implied by the discourses Bathmaker refers to. For example, Wheelahan, in her (2007) Bernsteinian analysis of knowledge and vocational education, argued that VET students should be able to access disciplinary boundaries and have the capacity to negotiate those boundaries in their practice. CBT, she argues, renders those boundaries invisible, and denies VET students access to forms of knowledge conferred on 'those students studying elite professions'. Whilst Wheelahan described a professional/vocational binary, it is evident that contemporary forms of teacher training, particularly for the FE sector, have far more in common with the VET programmes she discusses than with the 'elite professions', not least in terms of the curriculum which FE teachers access. More recently, Winch (2015, p. 168), discussing the practical abilities of the professional, argues that attempting to classify these forms of knowledge according to contemporary narrow concepts of skill is 'hopeless'. Instead, he advocates the development of a framework which can offer 'an adequate account of practical knowledge which comprehends independence in action and judgement, as well as character elements of know-how, including the moral dimension of action, and relates these different elements', something which is consistent with the disciplinary knowledge advocated by Wheelahan, and which, as Bathmaker argues, is consistent with questions of equity and justice. The absence of powerful knowledge on which FE teachers can build their practice as teachers, also begs questions about their ability to facilitate their own students to access knowledge which will enable them to take a full role in civic society, and about ways in which they might come to develop more democratic notions of professionalism.

It is apparent that more democratic notions of professionalism, which emphasise concepts of agency and autonomy, are in tension with the notions of professionalism inscribed in the discourses of competency-based frameworks of teacher training. As early as 1997, Davies and Ferguson, writing about compulsory-phase Initial Teacher Education (ITE), raised concerns about a narrowing of the concept of professionalism where that notion was constructed within a competency-based framework (Davies and Ferguson 1997) (see also Davies and Ferguson 1998), arguing that this may contribute to a de-professionalisation of teachers. Concerns such as those raised by Davies and Ferguson have run in parallel with critiques which argue that, in an increasingly marketised and neo-liberal sector, in which education, skills and those teaching and learning them are increasingly commodified, more traditional concepts of professional have lost much of their meaning as professional judgement has become 'subordinated to the requirements of performativity and marketing' (Ball 2003, p.226).

Despite the reductive nature of the curriculum, and the neo-liberal ethos which permeates education in both England and Australia, it is apparent that many teachers still develop those notions of professionalism which are more in keeping with Petrie's (2015) description (e.g. Jameson and Hillier 2008; Davies and Ferguson 1998; see also Evetts's discussion of professionalism in relation to Foucauldian concepts of legitimacy, 2013) and which are associated with more abstract notions of what it means to be professional focussing on autonomy and responsibility. It is possible that the process of acquisition of these more critical and reflexive understandings owes less to instrumental forms of teacher training and more to engagement with communities of practice adopting particular understandings or discourses around different aspects of the teacher's role, and which are more consistent with notions of the 'extended' rather than 'restricted' professional (e.g. see Hoyle 1980).

However, despite concerns about both professionalism and knowledge being well articulated across international contexts, both England and Australia continue to locate teacher preparation for the sector within a competency-based framework which fails to 'think beyond' narrow categorisations associated with prevailing concepts of 'skill' and 'knowledge' (Winch 2015, p.166) or to acknowledge the importance of scholarship and critical reflection (Winch, Oancea, and Orchard 2015; see also Bathmaker 2013) in the development of intending teachers. Whilst this sits uncomfortably with emancipatory notions of professionalism, it is consistent with the 'top down' managerialist and utilitarian concepts arising from the neo-liberal, performative discourses which have permeated education at all levels over the past generation (e.g. see Avis 2016; Ball 2015) and which, over time, have become increasingly shrill.

Conclusion

Such instrumental and reductive conceptualisations of what it means to be professional pose a number of wicked problems (Trowler 2012). First, they fail to acknowledge the agency of individuals who are trying to do 'a good job' (Jameson and Hillier 2008). Second, they constrain practitioners to a particular set of behaviours which can be associated with neo-liberal concepts of managerialism and performativity, whilst simultaneously denying practitioners the opportunities to develop and enact more democratic or emancipatory notions of professionalism, since the standards themselves lack any real conceptual underpinning. Thus, if, as Broudy (1972:12) suggests 'professional means theory-guided practice with the practitioner possessing both the how and why of the practice' and that no single observable behaviour is likely to be proof of understanding, since understanding is essentially a state of mind, the inevitable corollary of utilitarian professional standards will be a continuing and increasing de-skilling and de-professionalisation of the FE workforce (Avis 2007).

Disclosure statement

No potential conflict of interest was reported by the authors.

ORCID

Liz Atkins ⓘ http://orcid.org/0000-0001-9673-4428
Jonathan Tummons ⓘ http://orcid.org/0000-0002-1372-3799

References

Avis, J. 2007. *Education, Policy and Social Justice: Learning and Skills*. London: Continuum.
Avis, J. 2016. *Social Justice, Transformation and Knowledge: Policy, Workplace Learning and Skills*. London: Routledge.
Ball, S. 2003. "The Teacher's Soul and the Terrors of Performativity." *Journal of Education Policy* 18 (2): 215–228. doi:10.1080/0268093022000043065.
Ball, S. 2015. "Accounting for a Sociological Life: Influences and Experiences on the Road from Welfarism to Neoliberalism." *British Journal of Sociology of Education* 36 (6): 817–831. doi :10.1080/01425692.2015.1050087.
Bathmaker, A. M. 2013. "Defining Vocational 'Knowledge': Stakeholders, Purposes and Content of Vocational Education Qualifications in England." *Journal of Vocational Education and Training* 65 (1): 87–107.
Broudy, H. S. 1972. *Critique of Performance-Based Teacher Education*. Washington, D.C.: American Association of Colleges for Teacher Education. Office of Education(DIEM), Washington, D.C.
Clayton, B. 2009. *Practitioner Experiences and Expectations with the Certificate IV in Training and Assessment (TAA40104): a Discussion of the Issues*. Adelaide: NCVER, Commonwealth of Australia.
Clow, R. 2005. "Just Teachers: The Work Carried out by Full-Time Further Education Teachers." *Research in Post-Compulsory Education* 10 (1): 63–81.
Commonwealth of Australia. 2015. *Users Guide to the Standards for Registered Training Organisations*. Australian Government/Australian Skills Quality Authority. https://www. asqa.gov.au/users-guide-to-the-standards-for-registered-training-organisations-2015/ about-the-standards-for-rtos/standard-one/clauses/clauses-1.13–1.16.html
Davies, R., and J. Ferguson. 1997. "Teachers as Learners Project: Teachers' Views of the Role of Initial Teacher Education within England and Wales in Developing Their Professionalism." *Journal of Education for Teaching* 23 (1): 39–56.
Davies, R., and J. Ferguson. 1998. "'Professional' or 'Competent'? The Roles of Higher Education and Schools in Initial Teacher Education." *Research Papers in Education* 13 (1): 67–86. doi:10.1080/0267152980130105.
Department for Education and Skills/Standards Unit. 2004. *Equipping Our Teachers for the Future: Reforming Initial Teacher Training for the Learning and Skills Sector*. Annesley: DfES Publications
Education and Training Foundation. 2014. *Professional Standards for Teachers and Trainers – England*. https://www.et-foundation.co.uk/supporting/support-practitioners/professional-standards/

Elliott, G. 2000. "Accrediting Lecturers Using Competence-Based Approaches: A Cautionary Tale." In *Post-Compulsory Education and the New Millennium*, edited by D. Gray and C. Griffin. London: Jessica Kingsley.

Eraut, M. 1994. *Developing Professional Knowledge and Competence*. Abingdon: RoutledgeFalmer.

Evetts, J. 2013. "Professionalism: Value and Ideology." *Current Sociology Review* 61 (5–6): 778–796. doi:10.1177/0011392113479316.

FENTO. 1999. *National Standards for Teaching and Supporting Learning in Further Education in England and Wales*. London: FENTO.

Fletcher, M., L. Walker, and R. Boniface. 2013. *Summary of Practice Relating to the Development, Specification and Use of Professional Standards for Teachers across the UK and in Selected Other Countries*. RCU/The Education and Training Foundation Preston: RCU.

Gee, J. 1996. *Social Linguistics and Literacies: Ideology in Discourses*. 2nd ed. London: RoutledgeFalmer.

Gleeson, D., J. Davies, and E. Wheeler. 2005. "On the Making and Taking of Professionalism in the Further Education Workplace." *British Journal of Sociology of Education* 26 (4): 445–460.

Guthrie, H. 2010. *A Short History of Initial VET Teacher Training*. Occasional Paper. NCVER, Commonwealth of Australia.

Hoyle, C. 1980. *Continuing Learning in the Professions*. San Francisco: Jossey-Bass.

Jameson, J., and Y. Hillier. 2008. "'Nothing Will Prevent Me from Doing a Good Job': The Professionalisation of Part-Time Teaching Staff in Further and Adult Education." *Research in Post-Compulsory Education* 13 (1): 39–53.

Katz, T. 2000. "University Education for Developing Professional Practice." In *New Directions in Professional Higher Education*, edited by T. Bourner, T. Katz, and D. Watson, 19–32. Buckingham: Open University Press/Society for Research into Higher Education.

Kennedy, A. 2007. "Continuing Professional Development (CPD) Policy and the Discourse of Teacher Professionalism in Scotland." *Research Papers in Education* 22 (1): 95–111. doi:10.1080/02671520601152128.

Lemke, J. 1995. *Textual Politics: Discourse and Social Dynamics*. London: Taylor and Francis.

LLUK. 2007. *New Overarching Professional Standards for Teachers, Trainers and Tutors in the Lifelong Learning Sector*. London: LLUK.

Lucas, N. 2004. "The 'FENTO Fandango': National Standards, Compulsory Teaching Qualifications and the Growing Regulation of FE Teachers." *Journal of Further and Higher Education* 28 (1): 35–51.

Lucas, N., T. Nasta, and L. Rogers. 2012. "From Fragmentation to Chaos? The Regulation of Initial Teacher Training in Further Education." *British Educational Research Journal* 38 (4): 677–695.

Millerson, G. 1964. *The Qualifying Associations; a Study in Professionalisation*. London: Routledge.

Moodie, G., and L. Wheelahan. 2012. "Integration and Fragmentation of Post-Compulsory Teacher Education." *Journal of Vocational Education and Training*. 64 (3): 317–331.

Nasta, T. 2007. "Translating National Standards into Practice for the Initial Training of Further Education (FE) Teachers in England." *Research in Post-Compulsory Education* 12 (1): 1–17.

National Assessors and Workplace Trainers (NAWT). 2001. *Review of the Training Package for Assessment and Workplace Training: Final Report Stage 1*. Melbourne: ANTA.

Ofsted. 2003. *The Initial Training of Further Education Teachers – A Survey (HMI 1762)*. London: Ofsted.

Orr, K., and R. Simmons. 2010. "Dual Identities: The Inservice Teacher Trainee Experience in the English Further Education Sector." *Journal of Vocational Education and Training* 62 (1): 75–88.

Petrie, J. 2015. "Introduction: How Grimm is FE?" In *Further Education and the Twelve Dancing Princesses*, edited by M. Daley, K. Orr and J. Petrie, 1–12. London: Institute of Education Press.

Plowright, D., and G. Barr. 2012. "An Integrated Professionalism in Further Education: A Time for Phronesis?" *Journal of Further and Higher Education* 36 (1): 1–16.

Queensland College of Teachers (QCT). 2015. *Draft Professional Standards for Vocational Education and Training Practitioners V1.4.* Queensland College of Teachers.

Randle, K., and N. Brady. 1997a. "Managerialism and Professionalism in the 'Cinderella Service'." *Journal of Vocational Education and Training.* 49 (1): 121–139.

Randle, K., and N. Brady. 1997b. "Further Education and the New Managerialism." *Journal of Further and Higher Education* 21 (2): 229–239.

Robertson, I. 2008. "VET Teachers' Knowledge and Expertise." *International Journal of Training Research* 6 (1): 1–22.

Robson, J. 1998. "A profession in Crisis: Status, Culture, and Identity in the Further Education College." *Journal of Vocational Education and Training* 50 (4): 585–607.

Ryle, Gilbert. 1949. "Meaning and Necessity." *Philosophy* 24: 69–76. doi:10.1017/S0031819100006781.

Shain, F., and D. Gleeson. 1999. "Under New Management: Changing Conceptions of Teacher Professionalism and Policy in the Further Education Sector." *Journal of Education Policy* 14 (4): 445–462.

Shore, C., and S. Wright. 2000. "Coercive Accountability – The Rise of Audit Culture in Higher Education." In *Audit Cultures: Anthropological Studies in Accountability, Ethics and the Academy*, edited by M. Strathern, 57–89. London: Routledge.

Shulman, L. 1986. "Those Who Understand: Knowledge Growth in Teaching." *Educational Researcher* 15 (2): 4–14.

Simons, M., R. Harris, and E. Smith 2006. *The Certificate IV in Assessment and Workplace Training: Understanding Learners and Learning.* Adelaide: NCVER, Commonwealth of Australia.

Smith, E., S. Hodge, and K. Yasukawa. 2015. "VET Teacher Education in Australian Universities: Who Are the Students and What Are Their Views about Their Courses?" *Research in Post-Compulsory Education* 20 (4): 419–433.

Taylor, I. 1997. *Developing Learning in Professional Education.* Buckingham: Open University Press/Society for Research into Higher Education.

Trowler, P. 2012. "Wicked Issues in Situating Theory on Close-up Research." *Higher Education Research and Development* 31 (3): 273–284.

Tummons, J. 2014a. "The Textual Representation of Professionalism: Problematising Professional Standards for Teachers in the UK Lifelong Learning Sector." *Research in Post-Compulsory Education* 19 (1): 33–44.

Tummons, J. 2014b. "Professional Standards in Teacher Education: Tracing Discourses of Professionalism through the Analysis of Textbooks." *Research in Post-Compulsory Education* 19 (4): 417–432.

Wheelahan, L. 2007. "How Competency-Based Training Locks the Working Class out of Powerful Knowledge: A Modified Bernsteinian Analysis." *British Journal of Sociology of Education.* 28 (5): 637–651.

Williams, K. 2010. "Examining Education Qualifications for Australian Vocational Education Practitioners." *Journal of Vocational Education & Training* 62 (2): 183–194.

Winch, C. 2014. "Education and Broad Concepts of Agency." *Educational Philosophy and Theory* 46 (6), 569–583, DOI: 10.1080/00131857.2013.779211

Winch, C. 2015. "Assessing Professional Know-How." *Journal of Philosophy of Education.* https://onlinelibrary.wiley.com/doi/10.1111/1467-9752.12153/abstract

Winch, C., A. Oancea, and J. Orchard. 2015. "The Contribution of Educational Research to Teachers' Professional Learning: Philosophical Understandings." *Oxford Review of Education* 41 (2): 202–216. doi:10.1080/03054985.2015.1017406.

'Square peg – round hole': the emerging professional identities of HE in FE lecturers working in a partner college network in south-west England

Rebecca Turner, Liz McKenzie and Mark Stone

The professional status of further education lecturers has been widely debated and contested within the published literature. This article presents the results of a series of semi-structured interviews undertaken with a small sample of college lecturers working within a partner college network in south-west England. Regardless of the level of the higher/further education teaching the lecturers identities remain strongly rooted in their role as teachers and commitment to supporting learners attain their educational ambitions. The lecturers' identities were in a state of flux due to the dual demands of their employer (the college) and collaborating institution (the university). Their shifting identities may only be mediated through wider recognition being afforded to the role of a higher education lecturer working in a further education college from their managers, universities and supporting bodies.

Introduction

In 1997 Lord Dearing proposed a fundamental change in the delivery of higher education (HE) in England that would see further education (FE) colleges placed at the forefront of future expansion in HE (National Committee of Inquiry into Higher Education [NCIHE] 1997). Dearing cited the FE sector as being ideally positioned to promote the accessibility of HE courses to local communities. Although FE colleges have a longstanding commitment to the delivery of HE, for many institutions HE courses tended to represent a minority of their overall provision (Parry 2005). To support this expansion, in 2000 foundation degrees were introduced. Foundation degrees were intended to have either a technical, professional or vocational focus, consider flexible modes of delivery and encourage employer engagement (Higher Education Funding Council for England [HEFCE] 2000). They were to be delivered primarily in FE colleges in conjunction with a named HE institution. Placing FE colleges at the heart of the planned expansion in student numbers resulted in a renewed period of investment as colleges strived to create an environment for HE that would ensure students have an equivalent and appropriate HE experience to those studying at a university (HEFCE 2003a).

Traditionally colleges delivered courses that were approved, validated and inspected by external bodies. Therefore, the introduction of foundation degrees resulted in change in both institutional and individual lecturer working practices (HEFCE 2003a). Not only did they have to adapt to a new qualification, new quality systems and new collaborative partnerships with universities, for the first time college lecturers had the freedom to design courses in a supportive environment. It was also recommended that lecturers were provided with opportunities to undertake HE staff development activities, including scholarly activity and research to ensure that they had the current subject knowledge essential for their HE teaching (HEFCE 2003b). Through the expansion in HE provision, college lecturers gained new avenues in which to explore their professional identity.

Regardless of an individual's occupation their professional identity is viewed as being dynamic and constantly evolving as their career develops (Stronach et al. 2002). It is cited as being related to the culture of an organisation, social/professional inter-actions and an individual's self perception (Bejaard, Meijer, and Verloop 2004; Sachs 2001; Stronach et al. 2002). Research undertaken into the emerging professional iden-tities of trainee college lecturers (e.g., Bathmaker and Avis 2005) and school teachers (Bejaard, Verloop, and Vermunt 2000; Bejaard, Meijer, and Verloop 2004) highlighted the importance of the teaching context, perceptions of their role and professional expe-rience on an individual's identity. Equally the knowledge and skills individuals posses and the way they are expressed through their role also contributes to their professional identity (Stronach et al. 2002). Those working in the FE sector often enter teaching after establishing themselves as a professional within another sphere (Spenceley 2006). As a consequence, they bring to their teaching role a range of professional values and skills associated with their area of vocational expertise, therefore adding further complexity to their professional identities. This paper will investigate the impact of expanding HE provision on the professional identities of a group of lecturers working within four FE colleges in south-west England. Consideration of their professional identities will be framed through discussions of their perceptions of the roles performed by HE lecturers working within universities and colleges.

HE in FE provision in south-west England

HE in an FE context has been supported by the University of Plymouth since 1978. The University of Plymouth, through its partner college faculty (University of Plymouth Colleges [UPC]), is the primary provider of HE in FE in south-west England. UPC comprises a network of 19 partner institutions, 15 of which are FE colleges. UPC provides colleges and their staff with support for all aspects of their HE provision including quality assurance, staff development, administration and support for infrastructure developments. Since the introduction of foundation degrees in UPC in 2002 there has been substantial growth in student numbers, which has contrasted the national trend of foundation degree growth (Selby 2008). UPC's provision has grown from 6000 students in 2002 to 10,000 students registered on 296 courses in the 2007–08 academic year. These students are supported by 1800 lecturing and support staff.

HE in FE provision within the UPC network is highly variable in terms of longev-ity and size. Therefore, the experiences of lecturers delivering HE are dependant largely on the college in which individuals are working. While several of the larger colleges in the UPC network have a longstanding commitment to HE, in other colleges their HE provision is still developing. Colleges within the UPC network in which HE provision had already resulted in developments to support HE staff and students, such as investment in infrastructure or HE-specific staff development initiatives, were targeted to recruit volunteers to participate in this study.

Methods

To explore the emerging professional identities of HE in FE lecturers, a series of semi-structured interviews were conducted with lecturers working in colleges in the UPC network. College lecturers who had undertaken a UPC staff development activity were asked to contribute to this research. From those lecturers who volunteered to participate in the research 12 lecturers from four colleges were selected. Practitioners from these four colleges were selected as their institutions had a longstanding commitment to HE provided in collaboration with UPC. Therefore, in their college HE provision was well established which had included investment resources to support HE, HE-related staff development/support and the development of HE processes (e.g., graduation ceremonies). The lecturers were drawn from a cross-section of disciplines to ensure that subject-specific issues did not exert an overriding influence on the research findings. The interviewer asked the lecturers to discuss their educational and professional backgrounds, including how they became involved in HE teaching, their perceptions of the role of HE lecturers working within universities, and how these compared and contrasted to the role they performed were then explored. Discussion also took place about the support available for them to undertake the role of an HE lecturer. All the interviews were undertaken by one member of the research team who was not known to the participants. They were digitally recorded and transcribed in full. All identifying features were removed to ensure the anonymity of individuals and institutions involved. The transcripts were manually coded using the constant comparative approach; text being examined to identify comparisons and cross-cutting themes (Glaser and Strauss 1967).

Professional profile of the HE in FE lecturers

As a group the lecturers interviewed were diverse in terms of their educational backgrounds and professional experiences. Seven of the lecturers interviewed had progressed directly through the education system to university. Following graduation and throughout their professional lives, some of these lecturers had undertaken further study such as postgraduate qualifications and relevant professional development courses. The rest of the group could be classed as 'non-traditional students' in that they returned to learning as mature students. Two of the lecturers had undertaken their study while they were employed full-time. This had been achieved through flexible or distance learning to enable them to gain HE qualifications while balancing other commitments. The motivation behind these individuals' decisions to undertake HE again echoed the reasons mature students enter education e.g. to further their career or because of a life-changing event (Mercer 2007; Walters 2000).

Although four of the participants entered lecturing shortly after graduation, the rest of the group moved into teaching after they had spent time in another profession. This is well-documented within the FE sector due to the importance of vocational expertise to many of the courses (e.g., Bathmaker and Avis 2005; Robson 1998; Spenceley 2006). As with their entry into FE teaching, the majority of the interviewees did not necessarily plan to become an FE or HE lecturer. Instead they entered teaching because of a variety of reasons such as a need for their vocational skills/experience, through employer engagement or because they wanted a career change.

Entry into HE teaching

Of the 12 lecturers interviewed, half of the group were teaching at their college prior to the introduction of foundation degrees. Therefore, they had experience of teaching FE and Higher National Diplomas/Certificates. They did not necessarily aspire to become HE lecturers; instead it evolved as part of their natural career development, as they had been successful in teaching a variety of FE level courses and the next step was into HE:

> I suppose because of my vocational background (I entered FE teaching); I then started on a BTEC national level 3 programme. And I suppose I've been reasonably successful at that and it's sort of developed so that a few years later I then started teaching on HNC programmes...

For those lecturers who joined their college after foundation degrees had become part of their college's provision, teaching on HE courses was an accepted part of their role.

Roles and responsibilities of HE in FE lecturers

All of the lecturers were employed on FE contracts as is usual for HE in FE practitioners (HEFCE 2009). As with many lecturers working within the FE sector (Jephcote, Sailsbury, and Rees 2008; Avis, Kendal, and Parsons 2003), not only were staff engaged in teaching on HE courses, their roles had a considerably wider remit in terms of the levels, courses and subjects they taught across, but also in terms of more esoteric but essential aspects of their role that are often key to students' success:

> ...so I teach, I personal tutor and I spend a lot of my time on employer engagement....

Of the 12 staff interviewed, three taught solely HE and the rest taught on a combination of HE and FE courses. One individual also had responsibilities for courses delivered to secondary-school children and another had a dual role with teaching only a small part of additional commitments. Nine of the interviewees had responsibilities for programme management at either the HE or FE level. Programme management means that lecturers not only have to run the course and manage the associated paperwork, they also have some responsibility for activities such as marketing, recruitment, employer engagement and work placement visits. Furthermore, teaching to the non-traditional students that undertake foundation degrees also means that lecturers have to manage wider learning or social issues that are commonly associated with FE learners (Edward et al. 2007; Jephcote, Sailsbury, and Rees 2008).

The perceptions of the role of an HE lecturer working within a university varied. They all had HE qualifications obtained at different times in their lives, albeit through a variety of routes, and therefore they had an appreciation of the role performed by an HE lecturer working within a university. However, considerable time had passed since they had completed studies, therefore, they were concerned how much the 'student experience' and role of the lecturer had moved on since they were at university. These feelings were particularly acute for those individuals who had undertaken HE qualifications through alternative routes:

> I don't know for certain. I suppose it's interesting in that I'm expected to teach like a university lecturer but perhaps I don't really know what a university lecturer's role is.

Despite these concerns they all had definite opinions on the role of HE lecturers working within universities, particularly with regards to the contact they had with students and the support they received from their institution to fulfil their role.

The college lecturers viewed research as central to the role of a university lecturer and that their role as a researcher would be of primary importance over their role as a teacher. They viewed research as contributing to university lecturers' teaching and resulted in them having current subject knowledge. They also perceived that financial and practical support would be available from the university to enable them to be research active:

> I imagine that there is financial help, I imagine there is remission….

There was also a perception of the wider university ethos as being collegiate and research-focused. The college lecturers felt that this collegiately would encourage people to talk, share ideas and support the generation of new ideas. The lecturers indicated that this culture was encouraged by the level of autonomy which university lecturers had to undertake in their role. The college lecturers believed university lecturers could manage their own workload, which, owing to the limited contact with students, gave them greater freedom to undertake research:

> …they have allocated time for research, they've got allocated time and plan time they have at the beginning of the academic year if they are marking, for everything is planned ahead and structured differently, anyway that's my understanding.

In terms of university lecturers' commitment to teaching and their students, this was perceived as limited. They felt the relationship students had with lectures would be anonymous. Students would be taught in large groups and there would be limited one-to-one contact. This does not mean they felt that university lecturers do not support their students; instead they felt university lecturers would encourage students to function as independent learners:

> I just get the impression there is a greater volume of students and it is possible to have the same personal relationship?

The college lecturers' overall perceptions of the role of a university lecturer focused primarily on the responsibilities they have for research and teaching. These perceptions are reminiscent of the so-called golden age of the university lecturer where academic freedom prevailed and there was sense of collegiality (Barnett 1990; Light and Cox 2001; Nixon 1996). Clegg (2008) perhaps encapsulates this through her consideration of the traditional public perception of an academic which she viewed as originating from elite universities where departments were often populated by white, middle-class males. While a sense of collegiality still exists in many university departments, it is often viewed as being undermined by the changes that have taken place within the university sector (Lea and Callaghan 2008). This may also reflect the invisibility or ambiguity surrounding the role and subsequently the identity of lecturers to those outside of the university environment (Clegg 2008).

While they acknowledge the contribution a university lecturer's engagement would make to their teaching, in terms of them possessing current subject knowledge, they tended to view research and teaching as separate activities that did not overlap. This is despite the focus within discussions on the research–teaching nexus of the positive benefits of research–teaching linkages to the student learning experience (Jenkins, Healey, and Zetter 2007). Although a few lecturers did make reference to wider aspects of the teaching role they expected university lecturers to perform (e.g., assessing students/designing courses), it appeared that they primarily viewed the role of a university lecturer as lecturing to large cohorts of students. Today university lecturers are required to have an awareness of the pedagogical needs of learners, to design, market and manage programmes, develop and nurture postgraduate research- ers, while simultaneously remaining research-active, attracting research funds and publishing papers (Nixon 1996; Nichols 2005; Lea and Callaghan 2008). As with college lecturers, university lecturers are required to meet targets. However, rather than being focused on student attainment and retention they are centred on research activity through the Research Assessment Exercise (Elton 2001; Nichols 2005). Therefore, while the contexts in which university and college lecturers perform their role and develop their professional identities may seem worlds apart, there may be more similarities in the roles they perform than college lecturers initially perceived.

The role of an HE lecturer working within an FE college

In contrast to the perception they conveyed of the distance between university and college lecturers from their students, the college lecturers emphasised the central role students play in their working lives, with nine describing their role in these terms:

> I perceive my job as to create a learning experience through the course design, staffing and classroom interactions that allows students to maximise their potential and to succeed....

Owing to the socio-economic profiles of students attending FE colleges they viewed their approach to teaching HE as being holistic; not only did they deliver the subject matter relevant to the course, but also had to consider the specific learning needs of their students. This reflects the non-traditional educational background of the students they taught:

> So my experience with foundation degree students is that you are dealing with people who have to learn how to learn before they can learn what they are there to learn. They have to find the skills of reading, assimilating information, study, especially time management and they have to learn how to do all of that before they can learn about statistics, sociology, whatever it is they are there to learn from a subject point of view.

The focus on supporting students and the emphasis on skill development reflects the overall approach to teaching taken by lecturers working within FE colleges, especially their focus on the process of learning rather than the outcomes of learning as discussed by Hodkinson et al. (2007).

The majority of the lecturers felt that they delivered the same subject matter in their HE and FE teaching, but that it was differentiated through their expectations of their students and the assessment strategies they employed with their HE students to promote learner autonomy:

> My view is that we continue to teach subject matter that is now at level 4 rather than level 3 so it's a bit more involved, it's a bit more detailed... I think the way that we assess our expectations on students is different, I am expecting more research, more analysis to be presented.

They also discussed employing different styles of teaching with their HE students that would not necessarily be suited to their FE students or an accepted mode of FE teaching, particularly in relation to FE quality systems:

> I've just started doing some experiments using problem based learning as a method of teaching... and I find that I'm personally getting a real buzz from it because I see the students get a real buzz from it in terms of autonomy but also in terms of understanding the subject.

As well as promoting the autonomy of the learner, the college lecturers felt that the expansion of HE in their colleges had promoted their own autonomy as practitioners, which they had acknowledged as being a key aspect of the role of a university lecturer. Several individuals made reference to the sense of freedom or liberty in relation to their HE teaching. This reflected the opportunities they had been afforded to design courses, direct their students' development and collaborate with employers:

> I feel we are given tremendous amount of freedom to develop our own programmes to pursue what we feel we should be pursuing... in a way you've got far more freedom than you have if you run BTEC or national diplomas, you have to take them off the peg, even if they don't fit, if they don't fit the students, they don't fit the employers that you've got working around you.

For many this autonomy had contributed significantly to their sense of job satisfaction and in one case was cited as the reason why that individual continued to work within an FE college:

> It means that basically I've been able to choose what I teach in terms of the modules that are offered. Whereas if there was no HE and FE I would just be teaching hours and hours of repeated GCSE level classes and would probably be bored and be doing another job now.

The college lecturers all identified aspects of their HE role/practice which differed to the role they felt they, or their colleagues, carried out as FE lecturers. Therefore, within their colleges the lecturers felt that they were performing a unique role in relation to their university and FE colleagues. They felt their role as HE in FE lecturers relied upon them drawing on their expertise in supporting FE learners and integrating this with their perceptions of the role an HE lecturer should perform.

Comparing and contrasting the roles of HE lecturers working within universities and colleges

In relation to university lecturers, the college lecturers felt that their role involved a greater commitment to teaching and, subsequently, to their students. Generally HE in FE student cohorts are smaller, which the college lecturers felt enabled them to develop a personal and supportive relationship with their students. While this may be beneficial to students, this can create an extra burden as lecturers can often feel at the beck and call of students, something which they did not feel would happen in a university setting:

I think the different type of student is probably the biggest issue; they are more the sorts of students that survive better in a FE context which has different types of support.

The college lecturers also felt that the smaller student cohorts meant that HE in colleges was delivered in a different way to universities. They thought it was not appropriate to use lecturing with small class sizes and, therefore, an emphasis was often placed on group work. In colleges where larger cohorts of HE students did exist, the facilities (i.e., lecture theatres) were not necessarily available to lecture:

...the first thing that comes to mind is how some colleagues I know at the college would think that teaching HE makes it legitimate to lecture students, whereas mostly because we have smaller rooms like this, we have 20–25 or 18–25 people in a room therefore lecturing doesn't seem very appropriate.

A central concern for the majority of the lecturers interviewed was the requirement for college lecturers to teach across subject areas and levels. Of the 12 lecturers interviewed nine were teaching HE and FE. While the proportions of HE and FE teaching varied, HE and FE have very different audiences, teaching styles, quality assurance protocols and assessment regimes. Lecturers switching between HE and FE throughout the working week expressed a sense of being a 'jack of all trades' owing to the variety of roles they were required to perform. This switching between roles often left college lecturers feeling there was limited support from the college to specialise in their subject area. For example, this lecturer felt that there was limited support:

If you work here then I think you are expected to be able to teach anybody from sort of 14 going through to post PhD which of course you can't do that. I think you have to specialise but it's not recognised unfortunately...

Equally, this lack of support gave the impression that there was a lack of recognition from the institution of the wider implications of being an HE lecturer, as highlighted in their responses to questioning about opportunities for HE-related staff development, particularly in scholarly activity and research. The college lecturers were acutely aware of the importance of research, and the need for HE lecturers within universities to be research-active. However, they tended to view the research conducted by their HE colleagues working within universities as being predominantly 'blue skies' focused around knowledge generation. Within an FE context the college lecturers felt that it was essential for their HE teaching to have current subject knowledge and, therefore, they emphasised the need for HE lecturers to undertake scholarly activities such as conference attendance, professional updating and to be widely read:

Incidentally research... in developing academic knowledge isn't seen as important in FE as it is in a university. In FE the research is subject based research.

The support available for college lecturers to undertake scholarly activity and research was highly variable and seemed to depend largely on the area of college an individual worked. Overall the college lecturers indicated that the motivation for individuals to undertake scholarly activity and research relied primarily on the lecturer. It seemed there would be limited encouragement from college management. This does not mean that colleges were not prepared to support those individuals that wanted to undertake professional qualifications or attend conferences; generally colleges were forthcoming in providing financial support. Yet, in terms of providing a lecturer with the time, college support was perceived to be limited. The lecturers felt there was an apparent reliance on the part of college management for an individual to meet the demands of a course or maintain current subject knowledge in their own time:

> We have access to a range of CPD activities through the university, for example the xxxx programme. It just so happened it ran on a Friday, it was a convenient time for me, I applied and obviously could go. But I do think that the courses I've just been talking about, I chose to go on. The college has not said to me to do that and I don't think there has been any guidance from the college really at all quite honestly...

This may reflect wider contractual issues. College lecturers are employed primarily on FE contracts of 828 hours of contact time over the academic year, which equates to approximately 22–23 hours teaching per week. Outside of this contact time lecturers are expected to undertake the usual preparation and paperwork their FE colleagues are required to complete. There does not appear to be the time or space within this contract for those lecturers with HE teaching commitments to meet the wider demands of this role.

The fact that HE in FE lecturing staff are employed on FE contracts perhaps demonstrates the apparent mismatch of HE and FE systems that appeared to exert an impact to varying extents on all the college lecturers interviewed. For example, they made reference to the expectation of HE lecturers to take attendance registers, to participate in staff development activities geared toward FE teaching and the use of inspection or observation criteria that are suited to FE and not, in their view, HE:

> I think it's an interesting dilemma in that the college itself I think is very much focussed on FE where we have a lesson observation regime where probably after 15 minutes I'd be criticised if I'm still talking. If the students aren't actively engaged in some sort of activity I would be criticised for that.

> ...all of that is [e.g., staff development, IT] geared to FE. So we don't fit, we are a square peg in a round hole. For all of those kinds of things; our timetables are different; we don't fit with that, that causes problems if you teach FE and HE.

This mismatch in HE and FE echoes the findings of Turner et al. (2009), which highlighted the presence of a hybrid culture of HE in FE colleges, whereby college lecturers discussed delivering HE within the constraints of FE systems and protocols. It also indicates the target-driven ethos of many FE colleges, where activities need to be measured, monitored and assessed in order to comply with the management style of the institutions (Edward et al. 2007). This mismatch was taken by seven lecturers to indicate the lack of wider recognition or value attached to HE by their FE colleagues. They felt that currently there was a lack of support for them to perform the role they professionally felt they should as a HE lecturer, regardless of the environment they were working in. Yet, two lecturers questioned whether a strong distinction between HE and FE should really be made, particularly from the perspective of their FE colleagues. They felt that by addressing contractual issues or providing remission for HE teaching without similar changes being made for those teaching on FE courses could lead to an undermining of the role of a FE lecturer and create tensions between HE and FE. These individuals felt that while wider cultural issues regarding the support and identity of HE provision within their college did need addressing, these were not insurmountable. Instead they felt it was important that recognition should be given to the fact they were delivering HE within an FE context, and that HE in FE has very different purpose and audiences to HE delivered in universities:

> I think you have to accept that here HE is a small proportion of what we do, so as an institution we are not or probably neither should we be (HE focused), we've got to get FE right, it's what we do…

The emerging professional identities of HE in FE lecturers

The professional identities of those working in any sector of education have been acknowledged as being complex and dynamic depending on the conditions of practice, an individual's life history and social/professional interactions. Within universities lecturers identities cannot be considered solely through an individual's responsibilities for research, teaching and management, instead they are cited as being highly distinctive and framed in terms of professional autonomy and personal agency (Clegg 2008). The identities of FE lecturers are viewed as being equally as complex and sometimes fragmented owing to the vocational background of many lecturers for which an affinity often persists long after entry into teaching (Robson 1998; Spenceley 2006). However, unlike university lecturers, those within the FE sector are often viewed as having a low professional status owing to the overriding managerial ethos of many colleges and the expectation of lecturers to be agents for numerous education policies and agendas, eroding the sense of professional autonomy traditionally associated with the sector (Gleeson, Davis, and Wheeler 2005; Shain and Gleeson 1999).

The lecturers who participated in this research possessed the professional characteristics commonly associated with FE lecturers identified by Briggs (2005), whereby they were committed to supporting their learners achieve their educational ambitions. While their perceptions of the role of a university lecturer may be considered idealised or outdated, the role they viewed an HE lecturer in a university performing contrasted significantly with the role they carried out as HE lecturers working in FE colleges. This will have implications for their emerging identities as HE lecturers, and why we consider them as having emerging identities as HE in FE lecturers. Theorists of professional identity, particularly Bernstein, highlight the impact of physical location on an identity (Bernstein 2000; Beck and Young 2005; Day et al. 2006). The lecturers interviewed here are delivering HE in an FE environment. Socialisation and processes whereby an individual builds relationships with those performing similar roles or posses a similar identity, have also recognised this as being a fundamental aspect of an individual's identity formation (Bernstein 2000; Beck and Young 2005). However, as these lecturers stated, HE represents a minority of their colleges overall provision. In their colleges, despite investment being made to support HE, provision is normally contained within isolated pockets of departments primarily geared toward the colleges' FE courses and learners. Therefore, on a daily basis they have limited opportunities to meet other HE lecturers within their own college, or at the university. Indeed their engagement with the university is primarily associated with the partner college faculty and while this does provide a clear link to the University, opportunities to meet university lecturers are generally few and far between. Consequently they are developing and exploring their identities as HE in FE lecturers in isolation.

For many HE in FE lecturers working in the UPC network, participation in HE-related staff devolvement activities provides a neutral territory in which they can explore their emerging identities. Often such activities are facilitated by the University, but organised on the request of HE in FE lecturers, therefore they can offer the socialisation opportunities lecturers need and bring them together from across their college(s). The lecturers interviewed as part of this study considered engagement with scholarly activity and research as key to a university lecturer's identity, therefore as HE lecturers working in FE colleges they expressed a desire to have similar opportunities. Although in many FE colleges such opportunities may be limited, initiatives have successfully been implemented in recent years to promote scholarly activity and research (e.g., Cunningham and Doncaster 2002; Minty et al. 2007; Turner et al. 2009). These initiatives have acknowledged the positive benefits of staff engagement with research on the overall ethos of colleges and motivation of lecturers. Developments in quality assurance protocols (e.g., the Integrated Quality Enhancement Review [Quality Assurance Agency 2008]) and policies for the future of HE in FE (e.g., HE strategies [HEFCE 2006, 2009]) have reinforced the need for further support for engagement with scholarly activity. As the impacts of these developments begin to be felt by college lecturers, they should have a positive impact on their emerging identities.

The culture of these organisations and social/professional interactions also appears to affect the emerging identities of the lecturers. The college lecturers interviewed felt that there was an overriding sense of FE governance, which for them was an obstacle to the HE experience they were trying to create. This clash of cultures could have a considerable impact upon an individual's identity, particularly for those who are teaching across HE and FE courses as they are constantly shifting between cultures. This may result in individuals developing identities that are continually changing and in a state of flux. However, Stronach et al. (2002), in their discussion of the changing professional identities of nurses and teachers in the face of wider political levers influencing their professions, acknowledged the presence of split identities among teachers. While they viewed split identities as potentially causing teachers to juggle their own professional goals with additional external pressures, which may lead to individuals having frustrated professional identities, they felt it was unlikely and unrealistic for teachers to have one professional identity as this would lead to a loss of the diversity of experience and personal traits an individual brings to their role. This is particularly true for half of the college lecturers interviewed for this study, the majority of whom had entered HE teaching following a relatively circuitous route that included a range of other professional and vocational experiences that were not directly teaching-related. This also, to an extent, echoes the sentiments of those college lecturers who strongly felt that the uniqueness of HE in FE, and subsequently their role as HE in FE lecturers, should be celebrated.

Celebration of the role of an HE in FE practitioner has wider connotations relating to the recognition of college lecturers by college management, their FE colleagues, and also to certain external audiences and professional bodies. Again, Stronach et al. (2002) held strong views on the importance of professional recognition. They viewed recognition at the local and global level as being essential to the continued motivation and development of excellent professionals. At the college level appropriate recognition and remission from management needs to be given to ensure lecturers have the time and space to develop as HE in FE professionals. Equally, education policy writers need to recognise formally the emergence of the new role of an HE in FE lecturer which has resulted from the expansion of HE into FE colleges. Formal recognition of the role of the HE in FE lecturer by policymakers and supporting agencies may serve to overcome the perception from the college lecturers as being viewed externally as second rate to HE lecturers working within universities, which can lead to an undermining of their emerging professionalism.

Over time, as the role of an HE in FE lecturer is further developed and recognised, college governance and management structures will develop to ensure lectures get the support they need to develop their emerging professional identities. However, we are likely to find that while general traits of the HE in FE lecturer may be categorised with regards to the relationship they have with their students and their approaches to scholarly activity, owing to the diversity of professional and vocational experiences many FE lecturers bring to their role, each HE in FE lecturer's own professional identity will be unique.

Acknowledgements

We would like to thank the UPC lecturers who contributed to this study. We would also like to thank Ken Gale for his insightful discussions on professional identity issues. This research was supported by the Higher Education Learning Partnership CETL.

References

Avis, J., A. Kendal, and J. Parsons. 2003. Crossing the boundaries: Expectations and experiences of newcomers to Higher and Further Education. *Research in Post Compulsory Education* 8, no. 2: 179–96.

Barnett, R. 1990. *The idea of higher education.* Buckingham, UK: SRHE.

Bathmaker, A-M., and J. Avis. 2005. Becoming a lecturer in further education in England: The construction of professional identity and the role of communities of practice. *Journal of Education for Training* 31, no. 1: 47–72.

Beck, J., and M.F.D. Young. 2005. The assault on the professionals and restructuring of academic and professional identity: A Bernsteinian analysis. *British Journal of Sociology of Education* 26, no. 2: 183–97.

Bejaard, D., N. Verloop, and J.D. Vermunt. 2000. Teachers' perceptions of professional identity: An exploratory study from a personal knowledge perspective. *Teaching and Teacher Education* 16, no. 7: 749–64.

Bejaard, D., P.C. Meijer, and N. Verloop. 2004. Reconsidering research in teachers' professional identities. *Teacher and Teacher Education* 20, no. 1: 107–28.

Bernstein, B. 2000. *Pedagogy, symbolic control and identity.* London: Taylor Francis.

Briggs, A.R.J. 2005. Professionalism in further education: A changing concept. *Management in Education* 19, no. 3: 19–23.

Clegg, S. 2008. Academic identities under threat. *British Education Research Journal* 34, no. 3: 329–46.

Cunningham, J., and K. Doncaster. 2002. Developing a research culture in the further education sector: A case study of a work-based approach to staff development. *Journal of Further and Higher Education* 26, no. 1: 53–60.

Day, C., A. Kington, G. Stobart, and P. Sammons. 2006. The personal and professional selves of teacher: Stable and unstable identities. *British Education Research Journal* 32, no. 4: 601–16.

Edward, S., F. Coffield, R. Steer, and M. Gregson. 2007. Endless change in the learning and skills sector: The impact on teaching staff. *Journal of Vocational Education and Training* 59, no. 2: 155–73.

Elton, L. 2001. Research and teaching: Conditions for a positive link (1). *Teaching in Higher Education* 6, no. 1: 43–56.

Glaser, B.G., and A.L. Strauss. 1967. *The discovery of grounded theory: Strategies for qualitative research.* Chicago, IL: Weidenfeld and Nicolson.

Gleeson, D., J. Davis, and E. Wheeler. 2005. On the making and taking of professionalism in the Further Education sector. *British Journal of Sociology of Education* 26, no. 4: 445–60.

HEFCE. 2000. *Foundation degree prospectus.* Bristol, UK: HEFCE.

HEFCE. 2003a. *Supporting higher education in further education colleges: A guide for tutors and lecturers.* Report 03/15. Bristol, UK: HEFCE.

HEFCE. 2003b. *Supporting higher education in further education colleges: Policy, practice and prospects.* Report 03/16. Bristol, UK: HEFCE.

HEFCE. 2006. *Higher education in further education colleges: Consultation on HEFCE policy, HEFCE policy developments 2006/48.* Bristol, UK: HEFCE.

HEFCE. 2009. *Supporting higher education in further education colleges: Policy practice and prospects.* Report 09/05. Bristol, UK: HEFCE.

Hodkinson P., G. Anderson, H. Colley, J. Davies, K. Dimet, T. Scaife, M. Tedder, M. Wahlberg, and E. Wheeler. 2007. Learning cultures in further education. *Educational Review* 59, no. 4: 399–413.

Jenkins, A., M. Healey, and R. Zetter. 2007. *Linking teaching and research in disciplines and departments.* York, UK: The Higher Education Academy.

Jephcote, M., J. Sailsbury, and G. Rees. 2008. Being a teacher in further education in changing times. *Research in Post Compulsory Education* 13, no. 2: 163–72.

Lea, S.J., and L. Callaghan. 2008. Lecturers on teaching within the 'supercomplexity' of Higher Education. *Higher Education* 55, 171–87.

Light, G., and R. Cox. 2001. *Learning and teaching in higher education: The reflective professional.* London: Paul Chapman Publishing.

Mercer, J. 2007. Re-negotiating the self through educational development: mature students' experiences. *Research in Post-Compulsory Education* 12, no. 1: 19–32.

Minty, I., E. Weedon, K. Morss, and P. Cannell. 2007. Developing research capabilities in FE lecturers through practitioner led action research. *Practice and Evidence of Scholarship of Teaching and Learning in Higher Education* 2, no. 1: 64–78.

NCIHE. 1997. *Higher education in the learning society. Main report.* London: NCIHE.

Nichols, G. 2005. New lecturers' constructions of learning, teaching and research. *Studies in Higher Education* 30, no. 5: 611–25.

Nixon, J. 1996. Professional identity and the restructuring of higher education. *Studies in Higher Education* 21, no. 1: 5–16.

Parry, G. 2005. HE in the learning and skills sector: England. In *A contested landscape: International perspectives on diversity in mass higher education,* ed. J. Gallacher and M. Osborne, 63–92. Leicester, UK: NIACE.

Quality Assurance Agency. 2008. *The handbook for integrated quality and enhancement review.* Gloucester, UK: QAA.

Robson, J. 1998. A profession in crisis: Status, culture and identity in FE colleges. *Journal of Vocational Education* 50, no. 4: 585–607.

Sachs, J. 2001. Teacher professional identity: Competing discourses, competing outcomes. *Journal of Education Policy* 16, no. 2: 149–61.

Selby, J. 2008. HEFCE strategy for HE in FECs: Current developments. Paper presented at Higher Education Further Conference: The current and future direction of higher education in further education colleges, January 22, in Birmingham, UK.

Shain, F., and D. Gleeson. 1999. Under new management: Changing conceptions of teacher professionalism and policy in the further education sector. *Journal of Educational Policy* 14, no. 4: 445–62.

Spenceley, L. 2006. Smoke and mirrors: An examination of the concept of professionalism with the further education sector. *Research in Post Compulsory Education* 11, no. 3: 289–302.

Stronach, I., B. Corbin, O. McNamara, S. Stark, and T. Warne. 2002. Towards an uncertain politics of professionalism: Teacher and nurse identities in flux. *Journal of Education Policy* 17, no. 1: 109–38.

Turner, R., L.M. McKenzie, A.P. McDermott, and M. Stone. 2009. Emerging HE cultures: Perspectives from CETL Award Holders in a partner college network. *Journal of Further and Higher Education* 33, no. 3: 255–63.

Turner, R., P. Young, S. Menon, and M. Stone. 2008. 'In the sunshine': A case study exploring the impact of a CETL award scheme. *Journal of Further and Higher Education* 32, no. 4: 441–8.

Walters, M. 2000. The mature students' three R's. *British Journal of Guidance and Counselling* 28, no. 2: 267–78.

Professionalism, identity and the self: the de-moralisation of teachers in English sixth form colleges

David William Stoten

In order to understand the changing nature of professionalism we must consider how the work of teachers has changed in recent years and place this into its wider political and social context as the British State moved from a social demo-cratic model of the State to one based on neo-liberal ideology. Although much of the literature of teacher professionalism has focused on the school sector, we should recognise that the term also applies to the education sector as a whole and consider the changing nature of work as well as the wider social construc-tion of professional identity. The purpose of this paper is to interpret the development of professionalism in the sixth form college sector by drawing from the work of Critical Theory and Jürgen Habermas in particular. It also explores the views of teachers on how their professional identity and personal orientation to work are changing. In doing so, the paper will explore the power relationship that exists between teachers and the state bureaucracy, the interplay between practice and ethics and the re-professionalisation of teachers in an age of neo-liberalism.

The decision by the Coalition Government to recognise the transferability of professional status between the school and college sectors is highly significant. For teachers, it permits career cross-over between sectors. For employers, it opens up a new source of labour. For the state, it signifies how it is able to define occupational status and display its power over the education system. The issue of professionalism serves as a *leit motif* of the changing nature of education in neo-liberal Britain. The changing boundaries within teaching are also indicative of a convergence of differ-ent ideological traditions and the subsequent formation of a policy consensus within the political elite over change. This transformation of educational policy has taken place over decades and can be traced to the 'Great Debate' speech made by the Labour Prime Minister James Callaghan in 1976. The speech is seminal in the sense that it called for a reassessment of the economic benefits of education policy and opened up the debate between those who advocated 'economic instrumentalism' and those who wished to defend established 'liberal-humanist' notions of education. Although the debate was much more nuanced than two polar opposites, it did gener-ate discussion over the nature of the State and its methods of governability, the idea of an education market in which students were sovereign and the position of teachers. The election of New Labour in 1997 ironically signified the end of the social democratic model of education and its liberal-humanist values and the confirmation of the neo-liberal State with its emphasis on economic instrumentalism.

The changing nature of the British State

The State is the key change agent in modern societies. It possesses legal and political sovereignty over a defined territory and is able to implement policy through its bureaucracy. The period 1945–1979 was characterised by a relatively high level of consensus over the nature of the British State, its role and responsibilities. Moreover, the State sought to consult powerful 'peak' organisations when drafting policy – notably the trades unions during a Labour Government and the Confederation of British Industry under a Conservative administration – in what was a form of neo-corporatism. The period since 1979 has witnessed the dismantling of this post-war consensus over the State and its replacement with the regulatory State. The regulatory State is indicative of the move from a producer model to an agency model of delivery – in short, the State no longer accepts responsibility for delivering key public services, such as the utilities, but prefers to contract responsibility out to tender. Alongside this re-engineering of the public sector, the State has moved to a market-led vision of provision that is influenced heavily by thoughts of efficiency and efficacy. This shift to a market-led model of public services has important implications for the education system since it has engendered radical change.

Although the transformation of the British State is indicative of the shift to neo-liberal ideas, it has also been accompanied by repeated and far-reaching structural change within Government. As a result of the Next Steps initiative in the late 1980s, Government sought to redesign its administrative structure with the creation of Executive Agencies, such as Ofsted. The motivation behind this was both political and financial in nature. This move to 'agencification' meant that it was more difficult to hold these bodies to account since, unlike departments of state, they were not directly accountable to Parliament. Moreover, as a consequence of the 1992 Further and Higher Education Act, both sixth form colleges (SFCs) and general further education colleges were removed from local authority control and placed into the post-compulsory further education (FE) sector, under the aegis of the Further Education Funding Council (FEFC). This move was seen as removing colleges from the political control of local authorities and opening colleges up to the demands of competition. The FEFC was responsible for funding colleges and administering inspections until it was superseded by the regional and local Learning and Skills Councils that managed funding allocations and the Office for Standards in Education (Ofsted) which, together with the Adult Learning Inspectorate, conducted inspections according to a rigid set of criteria. Ironically, although the formal State had appeared to have been reduced, in practice its influences remained, and with it the rise of a bureaucratic technical-rationalist mind-set that determined the value of education. In 2010, this framework was again altered, with sixth form colleges being removed from the FE sector and tentatively placed back within the local authority 'family' but with their funding provided by the Young People's Learning Agency, which is itself to be replaced by the English Funding Agency in the near future. Throughout this period of flux, the power of Government agencies over colleges has been clear, even to the point of engineering the closure of institutions that were viewed as being unviable because of either performance or financial health. From a classical Marxist perspective, the fundamental purpose of the superstructure has survived the remodelling of the State, and with this its infrastructure of command and control. It is a theme that is developed more fully by Habermas and that will be explored below.

New Public Management (NPM), the quasi-education market and the implications for teachers

Although the State has reduced its level of involvement in many areas of British society, it has also engendered new forms of control over those who work in the public services, in what Ball (2003) describes as 'new forms of entrepreneurial control through marketing and competition' (219). This new mechanism for control is described by Ball (2003) as being encapsulated in three policy technologies: 'the market, managerialism and performativity' (215). The exigencies placed upon colleges are profound: they are expected to compete for students and funding, be self-managing and aspire to be outstanding and, as such, have engendered wide-ranging change at college level. For teachers, the reality of NPM is evident in the analysis of their performance through the annual lesson observation, analysis of examination results using 'value added' statistical models such as A Level Performance System or Advanced Level Information System and appraisal. The management of educational provision has, in effect, devolved to the individual teacher in new and very personal terms.

Although the Office of National Statistics categorised teaching as a profession in the census of 2001, it has often been viewed as a pseudo-profession by those on the political Right, who have generally defended the interests of the medical and legal professions. At the heart of the critique of teacher professionalism is the belief that teaching is a lower skilled activity than practising medicine or law, and that it attracts less well-qualified entrants. As Hoyle (2001) describes, this reticence to acknowledge teachers as professionals stems from two sources: the public's collective memory of school and their concern over teaching methods. Professional status is generally achieved through accepted claims to expertise, independent judgment and self-regulation. Although there has been a widespread public acknowledgement of subject expertise and experience of dealing with the classroom, teaching itself has resisted self-regulation, especially when imposed by the State as in the guise of the now defunct General Teaching Council and the unpopular Institute for Learning (IfL). The decision by the teaching unions in the further education sector to boycott the IfL is indicative of widely held disquiet about the model of regulation introduced by Government.

Professionalism is being redefined by Government, as has been recognised for some years (Bottery 1996; Beck 1999; Ball 2003), and reworked into professionality (Gunter 2002, 146) where teachers are required to adhere to the rules imposed by managers: being professional is increasingly becoming defined in terms of conformity and subordination. This development has important consequences for teachers, not least because it undermines their autonomy, but also because it impacts on their own value-system and self-worth. Fundamentally, being a professional is more than doing things well, it is also about being ethical and maintaining a self-identity. Ball (2003, 221) develops this analysis of performativity and the re-creation of professional self-identity into a discussion of a 'values schizophrenia' within teachers as they attempt to reconcile their own very personal view of professionalism with the need to conform to the prevailing organisational culture. The question of how teachers respond to the demands of site-based management is at the heart of this research and its findings will inform the discourse on new forms of professional identity.

Gleeson and Shain (2003) have contributed to the research on the changing nature of teacher professionalism through their work on compliance within the FE sector, highlighting the transformation of some college teachers into managers and others into those who are managed. It is within this context that teachers are regarded as being responsible for micro-management and playing 'their part' in running the College. It is a form of rhetoric that invites participation and loyalty but is designed to engineer conformity. In their study of middle management in the sector, Gleeson and Shain (2003) proffered a typology of compliance in response to change. The three categories of response encapsulate the reactions of FE teachers to a new set of values and notions of professionalism. The identification of 'willing compliance' (Gleeson and Shain 2003, 236) amongst some staff recognises the reality that, for some teachers, new forms of professionalism represent an opportunity for advancement that may correspond with their own career goals. For others, there is only 'unwilling compliance' (Gleeson and Shain 2003, 238) to the new contractual relationship that was imposed as a result of incorporation in 1993. According to Gleeson and Shain (2003, 240), the 'vast majority' of those surveyed reported 'strategic compliance' in that although they implemented change, they rejected the business ethics that lay at its centre. Such research demonstrates that although Government policy has been preoccupied with re-professionalising teachers by redefining their professional identity and responsibilities, this conditioning process has been not entirely successful.

The ascendancy of performativity and its associated notion of professionality have important implications for how we view teachers as professionals and what is expected from them as they are re-ordered into new forms of behaviour. Such a shift is mirrored, for example, in the training organised within colleges by management. In-house training – known as continuous professional development (CPD) – tends now to be focused on 'up-skilling' or 're-skilling' in order to perform a particular act or engender a mode of behaviour. There is a clear emphasis in such an approach on developing practitioner skills rather than engaging in any philosophical debate about their work and its relation to wider society. Moreover, it is often senior management that determines what constitutes appropriate CPD through financial control and choice of training. In an echo of Braverman's (1974) labour process theory on de-professionalisation through de-skilling and a lack of autonomy, it is a process that is controlled by management and not the individual professional.

Professionalism cannot be dissociated from the self and the ethical framework within which it is constructed. In recent years, the ethical treatment of workers has come to the fore as managers in the private and public sectors seek to demonstrate their 'corporate social responsibility'. Take, for example, the idea of developing 'emotional intelligence' and the promotion of 'well-being' health programmes, which were identified as areas for management training in some sixth form colleges. Such approaches are not simply indicative of a 'caring corporatism' but of the all-encompassing nature of organisational life. Critical theory approaches to ethics at work reject the idea of an abstract corporate responsibility and emphasise the need to establish ethical practice at both individual level and that of wider society

(Wray-Bliss 2011). The centrality of organisational life in constructing the idea of the 'self at work' is also apparent in the literature generated by critical theorists and echoes Habermas' ideas on the interplay between the system and lifeworld. In contrast to mainstream technical-rationalism and the idea of the uniform worker, critical theory asserts that there are many dimensions to the 'self at work'. For critical theorists, management control is exercised in both identity formation and cultural reproduction and works to re-engineer human behaviour, professional identity and self-worth (Thomas 2011). Such a process of indoctrination is inherently complex and may involve individual complicity as well as some resistance, but it is nevertheless powerful and fundamentally unethical.

The relevance of Jürgen Habermas' ideas to the discourse of teacher professionalism

Critical Theory offers a powerful critique of the State and its policies. The origins of critical theory are Marxist in nature. Led by Max Horkheimer and Theodor Adorno, the 'Frankfurt School' of post-war German intellectuals sought to explain the failings of modern capitalist society in terms of alienation, reification and spiritual impoverishment. In *Dialectic of the Enlightenment*, Adorno and Horkheimer (1947) highlighted the bureaucratised nature of capitalist society and its impact on the individual. It also set out to offer a view of the future in which individuals were treated ethically. Jürgen Habermas has developed critical theory further and applied it to the contemporary context. In his pivotal work *The Structural Transformation of the Public Sphere: An Inquiry into a Category of Bourgeois Society*, Habermas (1989) provides a critique of the 'public sphere' as both an idea of human organisation and an ideology. Habermas is intellectually eclectic, drawing from Hegel's ideas on dominant cultural norms and alienation, Fromm's Marxist interpretation of the state and its capacity for propaganda and, most notably, from Weber's (1957) liberal critique of bureaucracy and its 'iron cage'. For Habermas, although modernity has restricted the capacity of individuals to express their views, there remains the potential to challenge oppression and encourage open debate that can lead to greater individual autonomy. As such, we can see that Habermas moved critical theory from the orthodox Marxian stance of the Frankfurt School and closer to a more pragmatic position that is aligned with contemporary social democracy.

The importance of Habermas' work is twofold. Firstly, it provides an interpretation of how contemporary society is flawed and, secondly, he offers a view of how the deficiencies in late capitalism can be addressed. Habermas (1989), in *Structural Transformation*, argued that modern societies are characterised by two spheres: the 'lifeworld' and the 'system'. The term 'lifeworld' is used to encapsulate social life: the family, friendships and other forms of informal social relationship. The term 'system' is used to describe the formalised mechanisms of social control that exist, such as the civil service and agencies of the modern capitalist state. Importantly, for Habermas, although the 'lifeworld' may be inherently conservative, in that it is involved in cultural reproduction, it is characterised by relatively high levels of individual freedom and collective co-operation. In contrast, the 'system' is typified by control and oppression. Habermas (1989) argues that the modern state has created a dysfunctional system in which individuals are denuded of their individual autonomy, with their ethical framework re-engineered in order to meet the needs of late capitalism.

Habermas offers then a theory of social evolution within which the ideas of distorted ethics and diminished personal autonomy are prominent. According to Habermas, contemporary capitalism creates new types of identity, which leads to a distortion of civil morality and personal ethics through a process of 'de-moralisation'. In addition to this assault on the individual's ethical and moral frame-work, Habermas argues that new forms of knowledge are created and imposed in order to serve the interests of the system. This thesis accentuates the role and power of the state bureaucracy as an agent of change and chimes with research that high-lights the transformation of the working environment in education but also the lexicon of management (Gronn 1993) that has resulted from changes induced as a result of Government policy. The self-assuredness that underpins much of NPM is not only based on technical-rational forms of knowledge but is also indicative of a particular set of values that are produced by neo-liberalism. For Habermas, although Liberalism was associated originally with the advocacy of individualism, it has become con-cerned with the subjugation of people to amoral instrumentality by the state.

In order to counter this 'de-moralisation' of society and the assertion of amoral organisational management, Habermas argues for a fundamental review of how we arrive at a view of the world and how we interact with others. At the heart of this imperative lies a call for the re-appraisal of our normative mental structures and moral consciousness. For Habermas, it is simply not enough to think about why we do what we do at work but how we do it, and what it means to us as professionals when we interact with others. Inherent within Haber-mas' argument is the idea that we need to understand others' viewpoints and arrive at some form of an inter-subjective consensus that is both moral and ethical. In this sense, Habermas echoes ideas both from the German hermeneutics of Hans-Georg Gadamer (1900–2002) and from the tradition of American pragmatism of John Dewey (1859–1952) and George Herbert Mead (1863–1931). In his *Theory of Communicative Action*, Habermas (1984/1987) developed this critique of the ontological and epistemological singularity of organisational science and called for true moral and ethical discourse that is designed to estab-lish a social order based on democratic self-expression.

Research methodology

The core challenges for any researcher are to establish what their focus should be, why they wish to undertake such an exercise and how it is proposed to be conducted and disseminated. For the researcher who adopts a Habermasian methodology, the research tools used are conditioned by the particular philosophical and socio-politi-cal position taken by the researcher. In contrast to positivist philosophy and research methodologies, a Habermasian researcher rejects the objectivist view of knowledge and values-free research. For Habermas, all knowledge is the consequence of social construction and is open to competing 'validity claims', which reflect differing positions in contemporary society. Habermas therefore offers a critique of positivist epistemology but rejects Postmodernism in accepting ontological realism. For Hab-ermas, there is a reality to human existence and it is characterised by social and political inequality. Given the emancipatory imperative inherent within critical the-ory, and the accusations that Postmodernism has undermined the philosophical certitude of the Left, this realist approach is consistent with Habermas' political stance.

Although critical theory has been criticised by positivist researchers as prioritising theory over empirical evidence and lacking suitable criteria to evaluate research, one should understand that critical theory adopts a different philosophical and methodological position from positivism, and that it should be judged on its own terms. Habermas offers us a correspondence theory of knowledge formation and truth in which dominant ideas permeate society and distort its values. This domination of our social discourse by certain interests, notably the state and its bureaucracy, establishes an orthodoxy of language and mind-set. For Habermas, we must move towards a situation where free and open debate is encouraged and where competing 'validity claims' to truth can be heard. According to Habermas, such an intersubjective process of dialogue would ultimately lead to a rational consensus and democratic coherence. This position can be criticised from a pragmatic perspective – how do we construct such a process and how could it be managed in the long term? The answer would, of course, be found in a fundamental change in late capitalist society, and one that is at the heart of critical theory.

This paper aims to counter criticism of critical theory by offering some empirical evidence. In eliciting the views of teachers, this research investigation aimed to uncover asymmetrical relations within colleges and empower teachers to express their opinion. The research exercise involved 53 teachers in total from three SFCs, one in the north and two in the south of England. The research methodology took place in three phases and adopted mixed methods, involving a pilot questionnaire, a follow-up questionnaire and a research discussion. The first phase used a brief questionnaire that generated responses to a series of 20 questions that related to four core themes: the idea of teacher professionalism, the power of the State, the practice of teacher daily work and the impact of NPM and corporate identity. The questionnaire was given to a purposive sample of 20 main scale teachers and middle management in one institution, but not to senior managers. As this research was principally concerned with the impact of NPM on teacher professionalism and teachers' responses to this, it was decided that it would not be appropriate to elicit the positions taken by senior managers. Each of the 20 statements on the questionnaire was framed positively, such as 'I believe that teachers have a set of professional ethics' (statement 3), 'I believe that I can organise my own work' (statement 8), 'I believe that teaching should be regarded as a profession' (statement 9), 'Central Government policies reflect a wish to engage teachers in policy-making' (statement 16) and 'I think that Government and the teaching profession share the same values over education' (statement 18), and informants were asked to agree or disagree with the statement. The aim behind this questionnaire was to tease out views on how autonomous teachers felt and how they viewed possible constraints on their professional practice. The data generated could be used to show how teachers supported each of the statements and, in doing so, their overall view on their profession status.

This research was developed further in phase two, where a typology of identities was created to encapsulate the views of teachers. A second questionnaire expanded on the pilot questionnaire and sought to explore the degree to which teachers identified with the typology offered in this paper. Ideal types are useful in offering a collective label to a range of views that share some coherence but cannot be viewed in terms of absolutes and are open to criticism. Nevertheless, this approach can be useful in reflecting generalised positions and generating further lines of ethnographic enquiry. Such an approach has been used by Gleeson and Shain (2003), in which they offer a typology related to forms of compliance, and Page (2011), who presented a typology of management drawn from religious affiliation. The idealised types adopted herein were taken from the history of revolutionary Russia in order to present a range of possible viewpoints. The four idealised types offered are: Ideologue – an enthusiastic advocate of the current system, Intellectual dissident – a principled objector, The young pioneer – the opportunistic careerist, and Subjugated worker – the disillusioned and disempowered teacher. The questionnaire did not use these terms explicitly but presented associated descriptors that sought to elicit a response from teachers. Their response could serve to generate central themes for the subsequent discussion.

Habermas' emphasis on the co-construction of knowledge and the importance of inter-subjectivity is reflected in phase three of the research, which sought to establish an 'ideal speech situation'. The purpose of the 'research conversation' was to elicit teachers' views and the trajectory of the conversation was entirely unstructured, with the participant often leading the discussion and generating points. Since there is very little research published on SFCs (excepting Lumby [2002, 2003]), and even less from a critical perspective, the focus for the research had to establish whether there was any linkage between the ideas generated by critical theory and the empirical data. Finally, in line with mainstream critical theory methodology, some personal reflexion by the researcher on the research process itself was required. It was not only important to recognise the ethical context to their involvement and respect the views of research participants, but also to ensure their anonymity.

Research findings and discussion

The pilot and full questionnaires

The pilot questionnaire produced interesting data with clear differences in responses. The questionnaire was designed with five statements associated with each of the four key issues identified in the research methodology. It was therefore possible to discern teachers' views through an analysis of the levels of support for each statement. It is clear from Figure 1 that statements 3, 8, 9 and 15 generated the highest levels of agreement and that statements 16 and 18 generated the least amount of agreement.

The most positive response related to professional identity: it was clear with an average of 4.4 from a possible maximum of 5.0, that the vast majority felt that

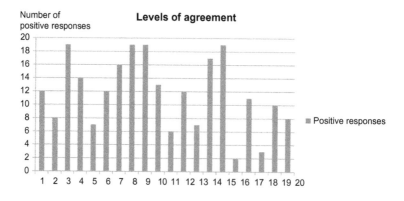

Figure 1. The level of agreement with the pilot questionnaire's 20 statements.

teaching was a principled and valued profession. This was followed by the key issue of autonomy, with an average of 3.55. It was evident that the majority of teachers felt that they possessed some degree of freedom to teach in the manner they believed appropriate. The lower level of agreement related to views of the State and Government policy, with an average of 1.65, and corporate management, with an average of 2.55. This set of data, albeit on a relatively small scale, suggests that there is some degree of empirical evidence to support critical approaches to educational policy.

The expanded questionnaire, based on the pilot, produced very similar data. Figure 2 describes the data generated from the full questionnaire. In terms of levels of agreement, statements 15, 3, 8 and 9 generated most positive responses, with 14 close behind. The lowest levels of agreement were generated by the responses to statements 16, 18, 13, 5 and 11. Again, as in the pilot, statements 16 and 18 generated the least amount of agreement. In general, this total was very similar to the earlier set of data and suggests some generalisability of the findings is possible. The aggregated data suggests that with an average level of agreement of 4.34 out of a maximum of 5.0, participants identified teaching as a profession with a discernible set of values and standards. Teacher autonomy also scored highly, with an average of 3.74, suggesting that the majority felt able to practise their skills without excessive interference. In contrast, with an average score of 1.39 and 2.38, respectively, the role and impact of the state and corporate management generated much lower levels of agreement. Taken together, this data would appear to provide empirical evidence to support a critical perspective on Government policy and its implementation at institutional level.

In contrast to the first part of the questionnaire, the lowest average score on the second part reflected the greatest level of identification on behalf of teachers. The data suggests that, with an average score of 1.33 out of a maximum score of 4.0, the 'Intellectual dissident' (statement 2) was the most common ideal type identified by participants. The Ideologue (statement 1), with an average of 3.21, was identified least of all by teachers. The Young pioneer (statement 3), with an average score of

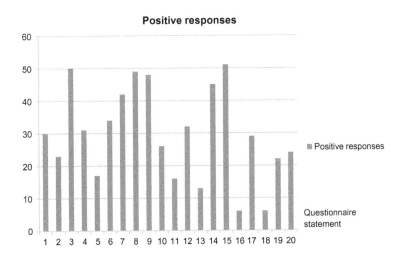

Figure 2.   The level of agreement with the full questionnaire's statements.

2.76, and the Subjugated worker (statement 4), with 2.70, were remarkably similar, suggesting that roughly equal numbers of teachers thought positively or negatively about their individual career prospects. This part of the full questionnaire highlights the relatively high levels of dissatisfaction within the teaching profession with the drift of Government policy and relatively little identification with its ideological agenda.

Teachers' views articulated in the research conversation

Comments made by teachers during the 'research conversation' varied with some support for the need for change but a clear majority expressed some degree of alienation with the current system.

One teacher thought that:

> Change is inevitable, in SFCs same as anywhere else. There are opportunities for career progression in the larger colleges as well as the smaller ones. (Male teacher, 55+, with some responsibility, 27 years of teaching experience)

Another thought:

> The teaching profession will always need to change to keep up to date with the demands from society – although we do tend to circulate every 10 years and then given a new title. (Female main scale teacher, no responsibility, aged 36–45, 13 years of teaching experience)

And another felt that:

> Change can be good and necessary, yet not necessarily in the manner they are, a business like mind is an attribute but ought not to be the leading emphasis – we are a life opportunity. I do not pioneer change as too much can reduce wisdom of time. I do feel disempowered. (Female, main scale teacher, aged 36–45, 16 years of teaching experience)

One teacher seemed to epitomise the idealised 'Intellectual dissident' offered in the typology:

> Under the influence of business ethics, education now tends to treat individuals as units of production, measuring their and the system's own worth in terms of usefulness, economic productivity, etc., paying mere lip service to any broader mission statements that promise to integrate a wider/deeper range of human values. Modern education is underpinned by a radically flawed philosophical anthropology to the extent that man is valued ultimately in terms of his/her value to the state rather than as an irreducible subject of unique dignity whose inalienable rights and identity find their ultimate justification in some transcendent ground of being. From this mistaken philosophy are derived systems and policies that favour a client-centred approach to education, favouring the practical over the cultural, the productive and utilitarian over the spiritual. An endless mathematical quantifying of achievements and targets, that is ultimately profoundly disillusioning and barren for all concerned, both providers and recipients alike. In a world where, in the words of one former minister of Education, Charles Clarke, 'Education for its own sake is seriously dodgy', knowledge becomes a tool for improving my material conditions, increasing my purchasing power, rather than a shared adventure of discovery and mutual personal enrichment. (Male, main scale teacher, aged 46–55, over 20 years of teaching experience)

There were a large number of teachers who corresponded closely to the 'Subjugated worker' offered in the typology:

> At the end of the day I get paid to do a job, cannot always expect to do what I like, but feel that the increasing rate of change makes people feel less secure and adds to dis-ease which can have negative health implications on teachers. (Female teacher, aged 55+, with some responsibility, 30 years of teaching experience)

> Incorporation changed the college. I got upset with the way Government changed how the exams system worked. It's all knee jerk reaction what the state did – certainly in education. (Male teacher, aged 55+, with some responsibility, 34 years in teaching)

> Definitely compromised principles. I hated [the college] but winding down to retirement. (Male main scale teacher, aged 55+, 36 years in teaching)

> Teaching is not regarded as a high-status profession – salaries indicate this. By nature I am cynical of others' motives, esp. politicians. I am a cynical realist. (Male teacher, aged 36–45, with some responsibility, 13 years of teaching experience)

The findings generated from both the questionnaire and research conversations suggest that teachers recognise that their working environment has changed and is likely to change further. This investigation also highlighted the widespread belief in a professional identity for teachers and recognition of the impact of NPM on their work. Ultimately, such research raises profound questions about the relationship between teachers and the State and echoes Habermas' thesis on the power of bureaucracy and the alienation of public-sector professionals.

Conclusion

This paper has been concerned with providing a critical perspective on the changing nature of professionalism in SFCs. The value of Habermas' contribution to the discourse on professionalism and the role of the state is manifold. In combining a theory of communication with identity formation, and offering a theory of social evolution alongside a vision of progressive change, Habermas provides a developed theoretical framework within which to analyse social and political power. This paper has shown, albeit on a small scale, that educational professionals in SFCs recognise the changing ideological context to their work and the pivotal role of the State and its agencies in re-engineering their profession. This research suggests that although SFC teachers retain a professional identity, they are suspicious of Government policy and are wary of NPM and its agenda to re-professionalise them. Indeed, it is possible to construct a typology of identities that teachers adopt in response to Government policy. This paper also suggests that teachers are subject to a process of 'de-moralisation' in that their values and ethical framework are often compromised by Government policy and the shift to a business model of education. These findings echo research undertaken in the wider FE sector and are indicative of a fundamental dilemma for teachers – do they position themselves as a profession to oppose such change, and if so how, or do they accept that they have been repositioned by the State? This is an area of research that requires further exploration.

References

Adorno, T. W., and M. Horkheimer. 1947. *Dialectic of the Enlightenment.* Amsterdam: Querido Verlag.

Ball, S. J. 2003. "The Teacher's Soul and the Terrors of Performativity." *Journal of Education Policy* 18 (2): 215–228.

Beck, J. 1999. "Makeover or Takeover? The Strange Death of Educational Autonomy in Neo-Liberal England." *British Journal of Sociology* 20 (2): 223–238.

Bottery, M. 1996. "The Challenge to Professionals from the New Public Management: Implications for the Teaching Profession." *Oxford Review of Education* 22 (2): 179–197.

Braverman, H. 1974. *Labour and Monopoly Capital: The Degradation of Work in the Twentieth Century.* New York and London: Monthly Review Press.

Gleeson, D., and F. Shain. 2003. "Managing Ambiguity in Further Education." In *Effective Educational Leadership*, edited by N. Bennett, M. Crawford, and M. Cartwright, 229–246. London: Paul Chapman.

Gronn, P. 1993. "Administrators and Their Talk." *Educational Management and Administration* 21 (1): 30–39.

Gunter, H. 2002. *Leaders and Leadership in Education.* London: Paul Chapman.

Habermas, J. 1984/1987. *The Theory of Communicative Action, 2 volumes.* Translated and edited by T. McCarthy. Boston, MA: Beacon Press.

Habermas, J. 1989. *The Structural Transformation of the Public Sphere: An Inquiry into a Category of Bourgeois Society.* Translated and edited by T. Burger. Cambridge, MA: MIT Press.

Hoyle, E. 2001. "Teaching Prestige, Status and Esteem." *Educational Management and Administration* 29 (2): 139–152.

Lumby, J. 2002. "The Management of Sixth Form Colleges: Implications for Leadership." Paper presented at the Annual Conference of the British Educational Research Association, Exeter University, September. Accessed June 16, 2006. www.leeds.ac.uk/educol/documents/00002438.htm

Lumby, J. 2003. "Culture Change: The Case of Sixth Form and General Further Education Colleges." *Educational Management and Administration* 31 (2): 159–174.

Page, D. 2011. "Fundamentalists, Priests, Martyrs and Converts: A Typology of First Tier Management in Further Education." *Research in Post-Compulsory Education* 16 (1): 101–121.

Thomas, R. 2011. "Critical Management Studies on Identity." In *The Oxford Handbook of Critical Management Studies*, edited by, M. Alvesson, T. Bridgman, and H. Willmott, 166–185. Oxford: Oxford University Press.

Weber, M. 1957. *The Theory of Social and Economic Organization.* Berkley, CA: University of California Press.

Wray-Bliss, E. 2011. "Ethics: Critique, Ambivalence and Infinite Responsibilities." In *The Oxford Handbook of Critical Management Studies*, edited by M. Alvesson, T. Bridgman, and H. Willmott, 267–285. Oxford: Oxford University Press.

The state of professional practice and policy in the English further education system: a view from below

Denis Gleeson, Julie Hughes, Matt O'Leary and Rob Smith

This paper addresses a recurring theme regarding the UK's Vocational Education and Training policy in which further education (FE) and training are primarily driven by employer demand. It explores the tensions associated with this process on the everyday working practices of FE practitioners and institutions and its impact on FE's contribution to the wider processes of social and economic inclusion. At a time when Ofsted and employer-led organisations have cast doubt on the contribution of FE, we explore pedagogies of practice that are often unacknowledged by the current audit demands of officialdom. We argue that such practice provides a more enlightened view of the sector and the challenges it faces in addressing wider issues of social justice, employability and civic regeneration. At the same time, the irony of introducing laissez-faire initiatives designed to remove statutory qualifications for FE teachers ignores the progress made over the past decade in raising the professional profile and status of teachers and trainers in the sector. In addressing such issues, the paper explores the limits and possibilities of constructing professional and vocational knowledge from networks and communities of practice, schools, universities, business, employers and local authorities, in which FE already operates.

Introduction

What constitutes professionalism in the further education (FE) sector, though high on the political and policy agenda, often remains opaque and contested among those on the ground. This paper, which has parallels with wider areas of public sector experience (e.g., Gleeson and Knights 2006), addresses the neglected field of FE as an arena of power and control, including its marginal status among statutory bodies and governmental agencies responsible for schools and FE provision. Drawing on case study material from an FE/higher education (HE) partnership in the West Midlands region of the UK, this paper focuses on the interface between *agency* (teaching and learning) and *structure* (policy and politics), in ways that impact on FE pedagogy and professionalism at a local level. Rather than reporting specifically on the findings from a discrete research study, this is a position paper that draws on data from two different projects dealing with 'live' areas of practice that are highly topical and contested for the FE workforce (i.e., the use of lesson observations and vocational pedagogy), both of which serve as illustrative vignettes of some of the key themes and issues discussed throughout.

This position paper argues for more robust forms of educational research and ethnographies that keep alive and make public the way practitioners build pedagogic cultures in the prevailing conditions of their work (Apple and Beane 2007; Ranson 2003). Following in this tradition, this position paper explores ways of reclaiming critical professionality in the processes of civic renewal and social justice that seek to move beyond the limits of market reform and call into question the so-called efficiency of marketisation. A key question turns on the way educational research critically engages with knowledge-making practices, rather than reporting the news (Shore and Butler 2012).

The research involves a multi-method approach, drawing on data from recent research projects. It focuses on two specific exemplars: (1) the use of lesson observation in the sector and (2) vocational pedagogy. The practices that these two exemplars refer to illuminate both the limitations and possibilities of reconnecting education reform to the ethos, nature and purpose of FE's traditional focus on meeting the broad, social needs of the communities it serves as well as the skills/economy-driven demands. This includes the prospects of improving teacher education programmes through 'criticality', incorporating the stories and narratives of the participants involved, sometimes in negative ways.

By criticality we refer to the ways in which FE practitioners and initial teacher education (ITE) tutors find ways of creatively interrupting a monistic skills agenda that Shore and Butler (2012) call 'the mechanic metaphors' and assumptions (204) that inhabit the lived experience (habitus) of FE practice. The dominance of a skills-driven agenda, ostensibly linked to improving employability, productivity and inclusion, has, in reality, come to mirror systems failure associated with the UK's low-skill, low-wage economy (Keep and Mayhew 2010). The market pulleys and levers that maintain such interventions (i.e., funding, audit and inspection) are supported by pathways and curriculum (emphasis on basic skills, competencies, learning styles, etc.) designed to keep teaching and learning in touch with a work ethic that is not working. Yet, despite the ever-shifting political sands of vocational education and training (VET) and FE reform, there is another parallel narrative that is perhaps more sanguine. Recent research centres, for example, on FE's increasingly important role in regional regeneration and capacity building at local level (Green 2012). Equally there is strong evidence of FE's engagement with the personal development of students. These originate in many stories and single moments that involve small, immeasurable and everyday incidents that help students change, gain confidence and grow (Evans, Schoon, and Weale 2013). This echoes recent research by BIS (2013) that indicates FE is more than a skills factory:

> Six in ten of all learners (60%) undertook training for 'non-economic' reasons: 45% of these learners said they did it to learn something new or gain new skills; 23% mentioned a personal interest in the course, while 16% of these learners indicated that they were undertaking the qualification in order to progress into a higher level of education and training. (7)

This questions the often deficit-based assumptions of FE teachers and learners as being primarily concerned with remedial courses, as far too simplistic. It is a view that largely ignores the diverse range of learner needs, motivations and interests in FE, within and beyond work and employer-led reform, that recent officially commissioned reports seemed so fixated on (CAVTL 2013; BIS 2012). While an important aspect of FE's contribution focuses on student wellbeing and job prospects, its diverse community and lifelong learning practice goes beyond a single economic purpose. In addition to conventional academic, industrial, agricultural, trade, apprenticeships and commerce programmes, colleges offer a wide range of provision, encompassing, for example, language and literacy, sport, leisure and recreation, offender learning, performing and creative arts, media and design, health and social care and childhood studies. Though the results often have positive economic outcomes, the measures of such success are invariably achieved through strong learning cultures rather than the imposition of prescribed skills or learning styles, for example (Coffield et al. 2008; James and Biesta 2007).

Changing teacher professionalism

The nature of FE teacher professionalism, though the subject of much recent research, is often misunderstood in the wider context of mainstream education. This is partly explained by divergence in teacher education between sectors, including historical divisions between technical, vocational and academic provision. By far the greater challenge to professionals working within and across sectors has been the de-professionalising effect of market and audit reform on teachers' work. More recently, attempts to deregulate teacher education provision, with a move away from College and HE partnerships in favour of employer-led initiatives, have raised the spectre of government and employer micromanagement of professionalism in the classroom and workplace.

Apart from a short period of mandatory teacher education reform, the ethos of FE teacher professionalism has traditionally been associated with occupational qualifications and prior work experience that historically eschews formal ITE processes, though this does not discount the existence of well-established ITE provision across a national network of higher education institutions (HEIs). While credential drift, associated with a significant expansion of academic-related programmes, has altered the technical and vocational landscape of FE/HE, many practitioners entering the field come from established trade and commercial backgrounds. Construction, business, engineering, hairdressing, catering, media and the arts are just a few examples of the industries from which experienced professionals have entered and continue to enter the teaching profession. Such expertise involves considerable prior work expertise and qualifications that often include experience of working with young people and adults of different ages and abilities, in a variety of work and community settings (Venables 1968).

At the same time, significant numbers of the students they teach and mentor come from similar backgrounds to themselves, which impacts on teaching and learning cultures (vocational habitus) in both positive and sometimes negative ways. In this respect, FE teachers' occupational biographies and transition into FE are less linear than those entering school and HE, though not exclusively so. The nature of entry into teaching among FE practitioners has become associated with notions of 'dual identity' – a term denoting how teachers describe their vocational identity in order of priority, that is, they see themselves firstly as an engineer, hairdresser or caterer and secondly as a teacher (Orr and Simmons 2010; Tipton 1973; Venables 1968). While such duality still holds strong, career entry into FE teaching is less clear cut today and is influenced by multiple identities associated with changing labour markets, programmes of study and cultural diversity, including life course transitions, redundancy and new beginnings. As James and Biesta (2007) have noted, although new entrants into FE speak of their altruistic desire to put their expertise and experience back into the community, others talk of 'sliding' into FE through casual and zero hours contracts that, by default, have become unofficial apprenticeships into FE teaching (Crowley 2014). Though such routes into FE are not new, the complex proliferation of fast-changing roles and job titles, characterised by the range of terms used, such as lecturer, tutor, trainer, instructor and assessor, reflects the diversity of the FE labour process. These roles also find expression in a wide range of often disparate academic, technical and vocational programmes that include on and off-site work placements. While part-time and casual working practices offer some degree of flexibility for teachers and managers, they also reinforce deeper distinctions between core (full-time) and periphery (part-time) staff (Gleeson 2014).

Recent research evidence points to continued, deep-seated differences between full-time and part-time staff by age, ethnicity, gender and disability, with men remaining over-represented in senior and technical staff roles (LSIS 2011). Overall, the data from the Learning and Skills Improvement Service Summary Workforce Report conclude that across FE, female staff are more likely to be working part-time than their male counterparts. It also provides wider evidence of homophobic bullying and under-representation of minorities in management and leadership positions, including the recent use of zero contracts.

Though exhaustive data relating to the FE workforce are not readily available, the picture remains one of a casualised and fractured cohort of the wider teaching profession, associated with restricted access both to ITE and to continuing professional development (CPD) opportunities. Despite FE's reputation for open access, social inclusion and 'second chance' provision, its staff and students operate in highly segmented and market-tested teaching and learning environments. It is puzzling, therefore, that three recent independent reports with a remit to improve the quality of teaching and learning in the sector (CAVTL 2013; BIS 2012; Ofsted 2012) make little or no reference to the narrow effects of workforce reform on teachers' work. A continuing feature of this process is that audit, inspection and funding-led regimes have become disconnected from the contested and often fragmented conditions – suggesting the official instruments of measurement are not fit for purpose.

In the sections that follow, we explore the implications of this process by looking at the micro-contexts in which teachers operate, resist and seek to reclaim a professional identity at work – though not always successfully. This is not an either/or process that can be readily understood in terms of restricted or expansive notions of professionalism (Lucas and Nasta 2010); it is also associated with identity around issues of resistance, power and contestation (Bernstein 1996), which we explore in the sections that follow.

Visible and invisible pedagogies of power: the case of lesson observation

One of the most hotly contested interventions to affect FE teachers in recent years is the use of graded lesson observations. Lesson observation has a longstanding role in the ITE, training and CPD of teachers, where it has been used formatively to provide feedback on performance or to model particular teaching approaches. It is only over the last decade and a half, however, that it has been increasingly appropriated as a policy tool with a new focus on teacher accountability and performativity (O'Leary 2012a). This focus cannot be de-contextualised from the wider proliferation of managerialism in FE as a whole, though the decision to hand over the remit for inspecting the sector to Ofsted and the subsequent introduction of the Common Inspection Framework (CIF) were significant milestones in crystallising this shift over the last decade. In this short space of time, observation has come to be regarded as arguably the most important source of evidence, along with student achievement, on which judgements about the quality of teaching and learning are based, both externally for agencies like Ofsted, and internally for FE institutions, as much of the performance data collection by them is invariably done with Ofsted in mind (O'Leary 2014).

Graded observations are summative assessments of a teacher's classroom competence and performance, typically undertaken on an annual basis and culminating in the award of a grade (1–4) based on Ofsted's CIF 4-point scale. These grades are then fed into institutions' quality management systems, where they are used in performance management as well as providing evidence for inspection purposes. Recent policy developments suggest that this reliance on observation looks set to be ratcheted up even further as teachers enter an era of heightened scrutiny and performativity with increasing demands for them to be observed more frequently (e.g., DfE 2010; Ofsted 2012). But what is the impact of this policy focus? Is it actually leading to an improvement in the quality and standards of teaching and learning in the sector? And what do FE practitioners think about how lesson observation is currently used? (See, for example, UCU 2013).

One of the key findings from a recent study carried out in the sector revealed how graded observations have become normalised as a performative tool of managerialist systems fixated with measuring teacher performance rather than actually improving it (O'Leary 2013). These quantitative performance indicators, or what is commonly referred to in the sector as the 'lesson observation grade profile' (i.e., a statistical data-set of how many lessons were graded 1, 2, 3 or 4 in any given year within the institution), have quickly become an established feature of college performance management systems and are accepted as valid and reliable measurements to compare overall performance year-on-year, forming the basis for the college's self-assessment for inspection purposes. In the comment below, Graham, the director of quality at a large college, accentuated the importance given to gathering and scrutinising these quantitative data on graded observations, as he was responsible for providing monthly statistical updates to his Senior Management Team (SMT) colleagues:

> On a monthly basis I report to the executive team on the current formal graded observation profile so the stats that they are looking for is the percentage of lessons observed that were good or better and then the percentage of lessons that were observed as inadequate and what we're doing about it.

Such practice is indicative of what Smith and O'Leary (2013) have labelled 'managerialist positivism', where the complexity of the teaching and learning process is superficially reduced to the presentation of quantitative performance data. Yet Graham, a senior college manager, was highly sceptical of its value: 'At the end of the year in our self-assessment report, we will report on the number of ones, twos, threes and fours and I think it's basically worthless'. Nevertheless, he conceded that, 'it's something that all colleges do at the moment because it's what Ofsted expects'.

One could argue that the hegemony of graded observations is perhaps a predictable consequence of successive neo-liberal intervention in teaching and learning over the last two decades and, in particular, the increasing influence of Ofsted. Since its involvement in FE, Ofsted's role has moved beyond that of inspecting standards to one of defining them, with the result that certain models of self-assessment are looked upon more favourably than others, as is the case with graded observations. Despite recent claims to the contrary that Ofsted does not prescribe a graded approach to self-assessment in the sector (Coffey 2013), Graham's remark that 'it's what Ofsted expects' strikes a familiar chord with many SMTs who are reluctant to veer away from current normalised models of observation for fear of standing out from the crowd, thereby leaving themselves more open to the critical scrutiny of Ofsted. The dominance of graded lesson observation is thus indicative of how Ofsted casts its 'normalizing gaze' (Foucault 1977, 184) over assessment practices in the sector and, in so doing, effects a form of panoptic control as the 'all-seeing' eye for 'standards' and 'quality'.

Normalisation can be defined as the adjustment of behaviour to fall into line with prescribed standards. Foucault (1977) asserted that 'the power of normalisation imposes homogeneity; but it individualises by making it possible to measure gaps, to determine levels, to fix specialities and to render the differences useful by fitting them one to another' (184). In the case of graded observation, the 'homogeneity' that Foucault refers to is imposed by the requirement for all teachers to demonstrate standardised notions of 'best practice' during graded observations. Those who are able to demonstrate this become accepted members of a homogenous community; those who fail to do so are identified through gaps in their assessed performance. The means by which such gaps are measured and levels determined is through a procedure that Foucault referred to as the *examination*, which 'combines the techniques of an observing hierarchy and those of a normalising judgement' (184). In this case, Foucault's *examination* is embodied in the annual graded observations that all FE teaching staff are required to undergo.

This process of normalisation is not, however, restricted solely to the mode of assessment, but permeates pedagogy too. Teachers are encouraged to tailor what they do in the classroom during their graded observations to ensure that they comply with prescribed notions of 'good' or 'outstanding' practice, notions that are largely determined though not explicitly defined by Ofsted. Terry, an engineering tutor with over 25 years of teaching experience, whose observed lessons had consistently been assessed as grade one over the previous 5 years, described with a certain sense of cynicism how he knew 'what boxes to tick' in order to get a grade one:

> I knew I was going to get a grade one because I knew what boxes to tick … if I used Power Point, if I included a plenary, if I proved that I was checking learning, etcetera. I could rabbit them off and I just went straight through a list. I got a one and it proved nothing at the end of the day. Ok, so I was told I got a one, but I just thought, 'so what'! The way the system is now is that if you know the rules you could be a crap teacher for the 35 weeks of the year but if you're good on that day because you know the game then you've got the tick in the box.

Terry's comments were indicative of how many teachers were aware of the need to 'play the game', especially given the high-stakes nature of these assessments and the potential repercussions for individuals and institutions alike (O'Leary and Brooks 2014). This in turn led to teachers spending disproportionately larger amounts of time in planning and preparing for these one-off observations than they would do normally. Invariably, the normalised models of 'best practice' that Terry and others like him were encouraged, and indeed expected, to adopt if they wanted to achieve a high grade, were cascaded from SMTs. As is the case with the recent development of comparative international testing systems for school children, such as the Programme for International Student Assessment, the search for 'best practices' has become the 'mantra' for teacher assessment and development in England, with 'comparison not only possible but imperative' (Kamens 2013, 123). However, rather than bringing about authentic and enduring changes in practice, this performative-driven emphasis has given rise to the creation of the 'showcase lesson', or what Ball (2003) has described as the 'spectacle' of an 'enacted fantasy' (222).

Another consequence was the reluctance for experimentation in the classroom as teachers feared being given a low grade and what that implied for the individual and the institution. Yet being prepared to experiment with new ways of doing things in the classroom and taking risks in one's teaching is widely acknowledged as an important constituent of the development of both the novice and experienced teacher (e.g., Fielding et al. 2005; IfL 2012). The advantages of observation models that prioritise development over surveillance are well documented. As Wragg (1999) remarks, 'good classroom observation can lie at the heart of both understanding professional practice and improving its quality' (17). Yet one of the biggest obstacles to the creation of such a climate in the sector at present would appear to be the issue of grading (O'Leary 2014).

Such is the level of significance attached to the annual graded observation nowadays that it has become an all-purpose mechanism that seems to have been adopted as the panacea of all matters relating to professional practice, and, in some instances, even replaced the appraisal process, as Terry recounts at his college:

Terry: … A few years ago with your appraisal, you had a yearly appraisal, of which lesson observation was only one part.
Researcher: Right, so that just formed one part of a wider process?
Terry: Yes, but the appraisal is now gone and we're just left with the animal that's called the lesson observation, which I don't think satisfies all the needs of the individual.

Terry's remark about the replacement of the appraisal interview 'with the animal that's called the lesson observation' not only draws attention to the increased importance of observation as a mechanism in the sector, but also epitomises what O'Leary (2012b) has referred to as the 'fetishisation' of the observed lesson insomuch as it has taken on the status of an all-encompassing tool with which to assess the current competence and performance of teachers, whilst simultaneously diagnosing their future CPD needs. A recurring theme to emerge from O'Leary's (2011) study, and indeed a more recent large-scale study (UCU 2013), was the perceived lack of benefit of graded observations to the CPD of teachers. Some said that college SMTs were the only beneficiaries, while others referred to internal graded observations as a 'tick-box' exercise that was more concerned with satisfying Ofsted than their development needs.

Wragg (1999) argued over a decade ago that the *purpose* of observation should largely determine how it is used. This would seem a fairly straightforward and uncontroversial statement, yet the boundaries between different approaches to observation and their underlying purposes have become blurred and contested. At the heart of these contestations lies a conflict between 'structure' and 'teacher agency' and the related notion of power and control that manifests itself in the sometimes paradoxical agendas of policy makers, the institution and its teaching staff. This conflict is epitomised by the way in which the developmental needs of staff and the requirements of performance management systems are forced to compete as they are often conflated into a 'one-size-fits-all' model of observation, with the latter prioritised over the former.

Formative approaches to observation such as ungraded peer observation tend to operate under the radar of metric-driven activity in many FE providers, with little evidence of the data generated from them being formally acknowledged or contributing to performance-related data. This does not mean to say, however, that they are any less valuable or have less of an impact on improving the quality of teaching and learning than those that seek to measure performance. Some would argue to the contrary, as indeed does Caroline, the vice principal of one of the largest colleges in England, who when asked whether she saw a particular model of observation as being more worthwhile than others, replied:

> I don't have any empirical evidence for my answer here, but I think if we could get a community of practitioners who actually valued the process of helping and supporting one another and would happily go in and out of each other's lessons and if we had daily conversations between teachers about what's working and what's not and idea sharing happening on an informal basis, not a formal basis, we will have won the battle. And the more formal systems you put in place probably militates against all of that because people then see it as a management driven initiative so we're not there yet but that's where we should be. In my view that would be the best possible environment, community of professionals, self-reflecting, sharing, talking, creatively thinking together and talking about their experiences would be wonderful.

Caroline's vision of a 'community of professionals' collaborating and sharing knowledge and experience on an informal basis exemplifies what we refer to as those 'invisible pedagogies' that play a key role in the ongoing development of practitioners and teaching and learning as a whole. In the case of lesson observation, such practice offers a credible alternative to current performative models of graded observation that currently dominate the sector. The extent to which such alternatives could or would sit comfortably alongside managerialist systems of audit and accountability that invariably value metrics-driven approaches to performance management more highly than qualitative alternatives is questionable. Surely though, as Caroline suggests, the way forward in maximising the potential of observation as a tool for improving the quality and understanding of teaching and learning lies in the adoption of an enquiry-based approach, where teachers are empowered to become active researchers of their classrooms. Until this is acknowledged by the relevant stakeholders, particularly policy makers, then the hegemony of graded observations, as an example, looks set to continue, and with it an impoverished understanding of what makes for effective teaching and learning.

Vocational pedagogy: the view from practitioners

As already mentioned, the recent Commission on Adult Vocational Teaching and Learning (CAVTL) (2013) can be seen as contributing to a government reform agenda that pays little attention to important contextual issues that shape the lived experience of practitioners – the lack of any critique of the impact of workforce reform as expressed in the Lingfield Report (BIS 2012) is an example. The foreword to the CAVTL (2013) report stresses the importance of the FE sector being able to 'develop programmes that address skills needs and wider learning for the sector' (6). A central focus throughout is on the need to identify and promote 'excellent' teaching and learning in vocational subjects and in attempting to do this, the writers identify four 'characteristics' of excellent VET, eight 'distinctive features', four 'enabling factors' and make ten 'recommendations'. The work of the Commission proceeded through the commissioners visiting providers, observing teaching, listening to learners, teachers and trainers, and employers and trade unions (CAVTL 2013, 12).

While the findings of the report are insightful, CAVTL is an example of a centralised and prescriptive approach to knowledge production for the purposes of developing FE in response to employer demand. We would argue that as a policy response CAVTL has two interrelated shortcomings. First, it potentially devalues the existing knowledge of FE practitioners by implicitly supporting an idea that there is a mysterious hidden principle behind effective VET that requires a group of people other than vocational teachers to descry, articulate and disseminate it. Secondly, in taking on this centralised role in knowledge production, it is filling a vacuum in a sector conditioned by managerialist cultures that have eroded the possibility of teachers engaging in their own relevant research to underpin necessary professional practice (Elliott 2006). To that extent, while seeking to promote 'dual professionalism', the Commission itself is premised on an ongoing structural process of de-professionalising FE practitioners, in which practitioner research is seen as incidental rather than fundamental to the identity of teachers in FE.

In the following vignette, we contrast the CAVTL modus operandi with that of a smaller-scale, localised research project: 'Building and sustaining partnership cultures in vocational pedagogy: practice, theory, leadership and community'. The ITE partnership from which this project grew sees itself as a 'community of practice' (Lave and Wenger 1991) – in this case, of teacher educators. This means that there is a conscious effort to blur the boundaries between FE and HE ITE provision. This 'blurring' is exemplified by the HE teachers all having a background of working in FE; by the use of sabbaticals for FE staff to work on the pre-service programme at the university; and by a franchising arrangement that attracts new colleges to the partnership through a strong level of engagement and interaction. The project used the CAVTL Report (2013), among other recent publications on vocational pedagogy (Faraday et al. 2011; Lucas et al. 2010, 2012; Skills Commission 2010), as a starting point for reflection and research with a group of FE vocational practitioners. This group was drawn from the colleges and institutions that belong to an HE/FE partnership delivering FE ITE in the West Midlands. The project had a number of key strands:

(1) to improve the understanding throughout the Partnership about what good practice in different vocational areas looked like through setting up subject specialist communities of practice across college boundaries,
(2) to develop the existing ITE programmes delivered across the Partnership to reflect this improved understanding and enhance the relevance and effectiveness of the qualifications for vocational teachers,
(3) to offer CPD opportunities for the practitioners involved, in particular through offering them the possibility of teaching on the ITE programmes as subject specialists.

A final research strand that ran through the project centred on a multi-method approach to gathering data about vocational pedagogy through a series of five full- and half-day meetings in which participants took part in discussions around how they got into teaching, how they learn best, their own barriers to learning and their current involvement with employers. They were also invited to reflect on the CAVTL recommendations and the theoretical models emerging from other literature.

The community of practice (CoP) concept was also used as a primary concept in the research project. The idea was to facilitate the establishment of a number of subject specialist communities of teachers from across colleges in the region. Nineteen FE practitioners from six subject areas took part, originating from eight FE colleges and four prisons. Participant involvement took the form of meeting together as subject specialist CoPs, both at the university and also in their workplaces. The project established CoPs in STEM (Science, Technology, Engineering and Mathematics) and Engineering, Construction, Offender Learning, Media Studies, Hair and Beauty and Health and Social Care.

The key findings that we share in this article connect with the idea that 'emotional labour' and pastoral work is a central though unrecognised component of the FE teacher's role (Salisbury et al. 2006). When asked to generate a list of the features of an 'excellent' vocational teacher in their subject area, the notions of 'care' and 'caring' were major themes that resonated across all subjects. The first participant to mention 'care' (a Media Studies teacher) explained how she took a holistic view of students that often involved helping them with wider pastoral issues. One example she briefly outlined involved dealing with one student's housing, benefits and shopping needs and how other members of her department characterised this as her 'mummying' the students. Rather than seeing this as a feature arising from an exploitative increase in the employment of women in the FE sector (Simmons 2008), we would instead view this as a response to funding-driven courses and the choices that teachers are forced to make by the prevailing managerialist cultures in FE. The point to emphasise is that the caring aspect of the Media Studies teacher's work was openly criticised by other staff. She was too caring in a context in which courses were there to be delivered and students were viewed as a means of securing funding. In that context, 'caring' was an untechnical approach. In this regard, we would argue that marketisation, managerialism and funding centredness have reduced caring in FE – or at the very least have marginalised the pastoral aspects of FE teaching – to little more than technical 'effects' that can be captured through student satisfaction quality assurance tools.

Furthermore, participants were not complacent or uncritical in their expression of the need for care. They viewed care as necessary but devalued. Their approach was always in tension with a dominant view of students as funding fodder. Other participants recognised the negative aspects of this labelling and asserted the importance of the pastoral aspect of their work. This echoes Hyland's (2006) commentary on the place of 'caring' in FE. In affirming a view that continuing reforms to vocational qualifications and marketisation are impacting negatively on students' experience, he suggests:

> There has never been a more important time to reassert the traditional 'caring' functions of FE which emphasise the importance of all students learning within the framework of close links between colleges and their communities. (8)

It is also important to distinguish what participants meant by 'care' from the 'therapeutic turn' that Ecclestone and Hayes (2009) have claimed is currently gripping education in England. This aspect of the work was not about conditioning students attitudinally for employment. Instead, the pastoral concerns here were a focus outside of any qualifications gained. Indeed, participants viewed the work as a neglected and devalued aspect of their work, being discounted by (some) other teachers and managers as it was time consuming but was not recognised in terms of college quality assurance or funding.

The centrality of this aspect of vocational teachers' work was echoed by an experienced prison educator working in Construction. He recounted dealing with a queue of heavily muscled inmates standing outside his office at the beginning of the day, all keen to see him to ask for help with a range of issues ranging from decoding lawyers' letters to discussing strained relationships with partners on the outside. In both cases, the vocational teacher regarded this 'caring' aspect of their role as a prerequisite to successful teaching and learning. This echoes findings in the literature around the fundamental importance of tutor–student relationships as 'the most important link in the whole process of further education' (TLRP and ESRC 2008, 6). For these practitioners, 'care' was not viewed as a detachable aspect of their practice but regarded as the cornerstone on which the features of an 'excellent' vocational teacher needed to be built; furthermore, it was seen as something that was increasingly pushed to one side by administrative and funding concerns.

Echoing a point made in CAVTL that a key enabling factor is 'a collaborative approach to accountability in order to empower VET professionals to maximise impact for employers and learners', participants expressed strong views on how managerialist systems of accountability failed to recognise effective VET where it connected to the 'growth' of students and abraded against self-generated models of professionalism. Amy stated:

> You are limited in what you can actually deliver and a lot of it can be down to [the college] because we are all so funding focused .... Programme Management Board is where people get told off for everything they've done. That's the best way of describing it. This colleague was defending a particular course. He'd lost three students off his course, 15 weeks into the course and all hell broke loose: 'Why did you lose these students?' In fact they had gone onto apprenticeships – one of them had gone into the trade and was still receiving training at the college. And to me, those individuals had gone on and 'Well done. Fantastic!' But no, the figures reflected negatively .... This is the stifling that happens at college level. Success should be measured by people going on to have a successful career.

This passage reveals that the student-orientated 'care' viewed by participants as central to their sense of excellence in VET is 'invisible' to existing quality assurance technologies in colleges. Furthermore, while teaching staff may maintain a 'clear line of sight to work' (CAVTL 2013, 9), where this cuts across college funding, cultures of accountability and blame have the effect of subordinating the interests of the student to those of the institution.

This theme of data-driven cultures in colleges as an obstacle to the flowering of effective VET and the sense of professional identity amongst VET teachers was a prominent theme running across data-sets. Rick provided a further example:

> We had three learners who went into employment and because it was after the six-week period, it had an overall effect on our success rates, and the overall effect of that

was that we came in at 0.9% below the national average. So instead of saying 'Well done!' we were put in … 'intensive care' – that's the term they use.

Rick's example demonstrates that the newly established 'Learning Programme' approach to funding – which privileges student retention over qualification completions – is as blunt an instrument as previous incarnations of the FE funding methodology (see Smith and O'Leary 2013 for examples).

Overall, the data provided from the project offered a very different perspective from that represented in existing literature (CAVTL 2013; Claxton et al. 2010) in that contextual factors were signalled as presenting significant obstacles to effective VET. Perhaps the most important contribution was the perspective of practitioners that skills development cannot be divorced from the life world contexts of students and that effective VET teachers strive to address educational goals within a localised setting while embracing the broader FE aims of social inclusion. It is perhaps unsurprising that this locally produced knowledge should provide a richer and more nuanced picture than the decontextualised and abstract version of VET that seems to be promoted by centralised discourses. This might best be explained through reference to two phenomena that have increasingly characterised FE over the last two decades. The first is the over-emphasis on quantitative data as a consequence of funding that has had the effect of engendering and then sustaining cultures of managerialism and performativity in colleges. This has resulted in the systematised privileging of quantitative over qualitative data and has had the effect of tearing away the contextual frame that is needed to understand college data (Lee 2012; Smith and O'Leary 2013). When complemented by the fabrication of data that managerialist cultures give rise to, the risk of reliability being compromised is magnified.

The second contributory factor is the maelstrom of policy that afflicts the sector – to the extent that no reform is allowed to bed down. The turmoil generated by annual changes to funding and curriculum prompted the 157 Group[1] to write an open letter to the incoming Minister of Skills in August 2014, pleading for respite:

> To do more at this point runs the risk of setting all this previous 'doing' up to fail. People … can only cope with so much change at once. Many of the reforms to date have received strong support from colleges, but time is needed to embed them. We hope that your arrival gives us a valuable opportunity for some much-needed breathing space to ensure the best success for learners. (Sedgmore 2014)

The welter of policy is fed by data, while at the same time generating more data in a sterile cycle. It is not difficult to understand how 'care' falls outside education when it is viewed in this way, as a technical delivery system.

What is concerning is that a defining feature of the terrain as identified in the project is barely mentioned in most policy literature. We would argue that by failing to highlight these phenomena while engaging with a 'best practice' agenda for workforce development, CAVTL may serve to impede rather than facilitate the enhancement of VET in FE.

Pedagogy, social justice and employability

If one effect of market and neo-liberal reform has been to separate FE off from its core business and values, as an 'alternative route' of 'second chance provision', another is the appropriation that successive governments have made in controlling recession and collapsed labour markets through the so-called 'skills agenda'. Since

FE incorporation, recurring patterns of VET policy and practice have essentially tracked rather than challenged the UK's low-skill, low-wage economy (Keep and Mayhew 2010). The subsequent plethora of VET initiatives both promotes and reflects recurring crises generated by market, policy and system failure. Recent OECD research (Green 2012) points to a 'tsunami' of policy initiatives over the past two decades that has restricted the ambitions of colleges, communities and local employers, in building infrastructural growth in the contexts and cultures in which they operate. Recurring themes from cognate research projects (e.g., ESRC: TLRP/ LLAKES[2]) identify five areas that have contributed to systemic policy failure that has impacted on FE, including:

- the use made of colleges as a substitute for employment and an extension of post-compulsory education,
- the restriction of college, community and employer partnerships, due to competition and the removal of regional tiers of strategic local government and economic planning,
- the increased reliance on outsourcing FE provision to private providers, getting students into work without checks and balances, on a payments-by-results basis,
- the dominance of corporate employer voice, demanding subsidies and tax breaks for participating at the selective end of the VET system and disadvantaging small and medium-sized enterprises,
- the persistence of skills over pedagogy at levels 1 and 2, maintaining a low skills ceiling that reduces learner progression.

While colleges and their staff are well-practised in mediating the vagaries of the market, their energy and resources have been channelled in diverse directions that have reduced pedagogy and professional development to second-order priority. The continuing effects of youth unemployment and weak labour markets have, according to Green (2012), dominated a skills agenda which in terms of its learners, '... is only part of the mix and not the fix' (59). If one consequence of this is to place limits on critical pedagogy and teacher development, another is the way it restricts colleges' potential as regional learning hubs, in the wider process of social and economic renewal. At the same time, Green's case study data portray FE colleges as significant 'bridging institutions' that address 'real world challenges', raising both the ambitions of employers and learners in the community:

> They provide bridges between employers and individuals ... in fostering bottom up innovation which focuses on the capacity of workers and companies to innovate and move up the value chain ... [and] can help provide the life skills for navigating not only the labour market but life in general. (2012, 60)

Alongside such findings, parallel research questions the prevailing view that the returns to public investment in FE are too low to warrant large-scale infrastructural funding and investment. Recent ESRC research indicates that under growing conditions of social polarisation, exclusion and uncertainty, FE has a protective effect in keeping young people and adults close to changing and volatile labour markets (Evans, Schoon, and Weale 2013). This role also involves the largely ignored process that supports productive adult transitions and turning points associated with learners and the life course, operating largely under the radar of inspection regimes.

The problem with audit and inspection cultures is, however, less to do with their existence than the way they misrecognise the conditions in which really useful knowledge is produced and how this also challenges systems failure and rescues lives (Gane 2012). As Rustin (2013) has noted:

> Audit and inspection are commonly seen as engines of standardisation and one dimensionality ... but need they be? Could forms of public accountability not be developed which are inclusive and democratic, and which were attentive to human qualities of service, rather than to their conformity to rules, procedures and outputs? (15)

Reflecting on this critique, Apple (2009) maintains that public story telling through research and practice has an important function in keeping alive the possibility of making public the successes of individuals and institutions contesting market controls over policies, curriculum and pedagogy. While alone such interventions may not be sufficient, Apple argues that a critical ethnographic dimension to educational research provides professionals with concrete policies and practices that will enable them to act practically in their own institutions, against prevailing models of surveillance and de-professionalisation. In support of this approach, both Elliott (2009) and Ranson (2003) argue that research-based teaching is becoming increasingly more compelling. It involves making public teachers' stories of building curriculum and pedagogy that embody Ranson's view of a reconstituted public sphere, based on difference, participation, dissent and social justice. This may or may not always relate directly to the acquisition of employable skills but certainly should involve interaction with students at a level that demands their engagement as thinking individuals.

While it would be inaccurate to say that mainstream educational research does not challenge or criticise the status quo, the findings of research are often overtaken by policy change and fashion or disappear through the ether of ministerial disappointment with answers they did not expect (Back and Puwar 2012). If really useful educational research is to transcend the immediacy of spot social knowledge generated by social media, it needs to engage with 'live research methods' that capture the different ways educational knowledge is constructed in the contested contexts in which stories are told. This relates back to the marketisation of the sector and the proliferation of knowledge production practices that are shaped by performativity (Ball 2003). The official discourse around FE that informs policy-making draws heavily on the largely unreliable data generated by managerialist/positivist cultures within colleges (Smith and O'Leary 2013) and is supported, it would seem, by the culture of performative knowledge production that currently underpins UK political life. Educational research that is locally co-produced by practitioners and researchers closely allied to local contexts has the ability to act as an antidote to this in the short term. We would suggest that locally produced knowledge in the current climate is necessary to restore balance against detrimentally centralised knowledge production practices.

While welcoming the recent focus on vocational pedagogy in FE, we are concerned that the emphasis on 'how to teach', learning styles and skills remains more closely tied to surface knowledge and inspection criteria than engaging critically with building capability that supports the needs and expertise of learners and teachers on the ground. The current freedom of the employer to make decisions regarding who to train, whether they are students or teachers, will undoubtedly lead to greater social injustices and failures in the VET system than exist at present. Reversing this trend through research and teacher education alone may not suffice. However, growing disbelief in the controlling effects of neo-liberalism in separating off pedagogy from its purpose and value is now raising pressing questions about what that connection should be, and for whom.

Concluding comments

While evidence from this paper indicates the nature and purpose of FE practice rests close to the surface of teacher identity, the tensions between practitioners being perceived as education workers or empowered professionals remain highly contested. Looking to the future, therefore, what can reasonably be expected of FE practitioners beyond the current contexts of their work? This question arguably turns on what not to do, given evidence of widespread systems failure in VET itself (Coffield et al. 2008; Keep and Mayhew 2010).

Broader principles of social justice are also at stake. A starting point might be an appraisal of the role of employers in VET. A re-evaluation is called for: first, of employers' freedom to define the VET curriculum and the right to curtail the entitlement of adults and young people to professionally trained and qualified staff; second, of their market rights to reduce the interactive and creative processes associated with the individual destiny of the learner, through standardised approaches that largely ignore the contexts and cultures in which VET learning takes place; and, finally, of major employers' demands for tax breaks, subsidies and government grants to train adults and young people in predominantly low skill, low wage environments.

A major effect of employer involvement overall has been to restrict learning and social mobility and effectively to reduce the funding of colleges and sector partners who are largely responsible for such work. In both social and economic terms, the private governance of public money not only endows employers with a voice without accountability, but also forms part of what Berg (1971) once aptly referred to as 'The Great Training Robbery'. While these considerations may not be the definitive answers to failings in the VET system, equally they explain the source of recurring dysfunctionality associated with successive laissez-faire political regimes that continue to tinker with the system without improving it. Without engaging the wider participation of partners in the FE sector in the production of contextualised and embedded knowledge, then sustainable improvement for staff and students is likely to remain elusive.

Disclosure statement

No potential conflict of interest was reported by the author(s).

Funding

The UCU (2013) report referred to in this article was a national project funded by the University and College Union.

Notes

1. The 157 Group is a consortium drawn from amongst the UK's largest FE colleges. It was formed in 2006 in response to paragraph 157 of Sir Andrew Foster's report on the future of further education colleges, in which he argued that principals of large successful colleges should play a greater role in policymaking.

2. ESRC = Economic and Social Research Council; TLRP = Teaching and Learning Research Programme; LLAKES = Learning and Life Chances in Knowledge Economies and Societies.

References

Apple, M. 2009. "Foreword." In *Changing Teacher Professionalism*, edited by S. Gewirtz, P. Mahony, I. Hextall, and V. Cribb, xv–xviii. London: Routledge.
Apple, M., and J. A. Beane. 2007. *Democratic Schools: Lessons in Powerful Education*. 2nd ed. Portsmouth, NH: Heinemann.
Back, L., and N. Puwar, eds. 2012. *Live Methods*. The Sociological Review Monographs. London: Blackwell.
Ball, S. 2003. "The Teacher's Soul and the Terrors of Performativity." *Journal of Education Policy* 18 (2): 215–228.
Berg, I. 1971. *Education and Jobs: The Great Training Robbery*. Boston, MA: Beacon Press.
Bernstein, B. 1996. *Pedagogy, Symbolic Control and Identity*. London: Taylor and Francis.
BIS. 2012. *Professionalism in Further Education*. Final Report of the Independent Review Panel Chaired by Lord Lingfield. London: Department of Business, Innovation and Skills. Accessed December 12, 2013. http://www.bis.gov.uk/assets/biscore/further-educa tion-skills/docs/p/12-1198-professionalism-in-further-education-final
BIS. 2013. "The Impact of Further Education Learning." Accessed December 12, 2013. https://www.gov.uk/government/uploads/system/uploads/attachment_data/file/69179/bis-13-597-impact-of-further-education-learning.pdf
CAVTL. 2013. *It's about Work: Excellent Vocational Teaching and Learning*. Commission on Adult Vocational Teaching and Learning. Coventry: LSIS; London: BIS.
Claxton, G., B. Lucas, and R. Webster. 2010. *Bodies of Knowledge*. London: Edge Foundation.
Coffey, M. 2013. "Graded Observation – What the Experts Say." Future of FE Conference, Guildford, UK, March. Accessed August 12, 2013. http://www.youtube.com/watch?v=tp4PoO8ArEo
Coffield, F., S. Edwards, A. Hodson, K. Spours, and R. Steer. 2008. *Improving Teaching and Learning and Skills Inclusion: The Impact of Policy on PCET*. Oxford: Routledge.

Crowley, S., ed. 2014. *Challenging Professional Learning*. London: Routledge.

Department for Education (DfE). 2010. *The Importance of Teaching*. London: HMSO.

Ecclestone, K., and D. Hayes. 2009. *The Dangerous Rise of Therapeutic Education*. Abingdon: Routledge.

Elliott, J. 2006. "The Impact of Research on Professional Practice and Identity." ESRC Seminar series: Changing Teacher Roles, Identities and Professionalism, King's College London, April 26. Accessed October 29, 2013. http://www.tlrp.org/themes/seminar/gew irtz/papers/seminar8/paper-elliott.pdf

Elliott, J. 2009. "Research Based Teaching." In *Changing Teacher Professionalism*, edited by S. Gerwirtz, P. Mahony, I. Hextall, and I. Cribb, 170–183. London: Routledge.

Evans, K., I. Schoon, and M. Weale. 2013. "Can Lifelong Learning Reshape Life Chances?" *British Journal of Educational Studies* 61 (1): 25–47.

Faraday, S., C. Overton, and S. Cooper. 2011. *Effective Teaching and Learning in Vocational Education*. London: LSN.

Fielding, M., S. Bragg, J. Craig, I. Cunningham, M. Eraut, S. Gillison, M. Horne, C. Robinson, and J. Thorp. 2005. *Factors Influencing the Transfer of Good Practice*. Research Report RR615. London: Department for Education and Skills.

Foucault, M. 1977. *Discipline and Punish – The Birth of the Prison*. Harmondsworth: Penguin.

Gane, N. 2012. "The Governmentalities of Neoliberalism: Panopticism, Post-panopticism and Beyond." *The Sociological Review* 60 (4): 611–634.

Gleeson, D. 2014. "Trading Places: On *Becoming* an FE Professional." In *Challenging Professional Learning*, edited by S. Crowley, 20–30. London: Routledge.

Gleeson, D., and D. Knights. 2006. "Challenging Dualism: Professionalism in Troubled times." *Sociology* 40 (2): 277–295.

Green, A. E. 2012. "Skills for Competitiveness: Country Report for United Kingdom." OECD Local Economic and Employment Development (LEED) Working Papers, No. 2012/05. Paris: OECD.

Hyland, T. 2006. "Vocational Education and Training and the Therapeutic Turn." *Educational Studies* 32 (3): 299–306.

Institute for Learning (IfL). 2012. *Leading Learning and Letting Go: Building Expansive Learning Environments in FE*. London: Institute for Learning.

James, D., and G. Biesta, eds. 2007. *Improving Learning Cultures in Further Education*. London: Routledge.

Kamens, D. 2013. "Globalization and the Emergence of an Audit Culture: PISA and the Search for 'Best Practices' and Magic Bullets." In *PISA, Power and Policy: The Emergence of Global Educational Governance*, edited by H.-D. Meyer and A. Benavot, 117–139. Oxford: Symposium Books.

Keep, E., and K. Mayhew. 2010. "Moving beyond Skills as a Social Panacea." *Work, Employment & Society* 11 (3): 213–266.

Lave, J., and E. Wenger. 1991. *Situated Learning: Legitimate Peripheral Participation*. Cambridge, UK: Cambridge University Press.

Learning and Skills Improvement Service (LSIS). 2011. *Further Education and Skills Sector: Summary – Workforce Diversity Report*, 1–26. Coventry, UK: LSIS.

Lee, B. 2012. "New Public Management, Accounting, Regulators and Moral Panics." *International Journal of Public Management* 5 (3): 192–202.

Lucas, B., G. Claxton, and R. Webster. 2010. *Mind the Gap – Research and Reality in Practical and Vocational Education*. London: Edge Foundation.

Lucas, B., E. Spencer, and G. Claxton. 2012. *How to Teach Vocational Education. A Theory of Vocational Pedagogy*. London: Centre for Skills Development, City and Guilds.

Lucas, N., and T. Nasta. 2010. "State Regulation and the Professionalization of Further Education Teachers: A Comparison with Schools and HE." *Journal of Vocational Education and Training* 62 (4): 441–454.

O'Leary, M. 2011. "The Role of Lesson Observation in Shaping Professional Identity, Learning and Development in Further Education Colleges in the West Midlands." Unpublished PhD Thesis, Institute of Education, University of Warwick, UK.

O'Leary, M. 2012a. "Exploring the Role of Lesson Observation in the English Education System: A Review of Methods, Models and Meanings." *Professional Development in Education* 38 (5): 791–810.

O'Leary, M. 2012b. "Time to Turn Worthless Lesson Observation into a Powerful Tool for Improving Teaching and Learning." *CPD Matters/InTuition – IfL* 9: 16–18. Accessed August 3, 2013. http://www.ifl.ac.uk/data/assets/pdf_file/0008/27890/InTuition-issue-9-Summer-2012.pdf

O'Leary, M. 2013. "Surveillance, Performativity and Normalised Practice: The Use and Impact of Graded Lesson Observations in Further Education Colleges." *Journal of Further and Higher Education* 37 (5): 694–714.

O'Leary, M. 2014. *Classroom Observation: A Guide to the Effective Observation of Teaching and Learning*. London: Routledge.

O'Leary, M., and V. Brooks. 2014. "Raising the Stakes: Classroom Observation in the Further Education Sector in England." *Professional Development in Education* 40 (4): 530–545.

Ofsted. 2012. *A Good Education for All*. London: Ofsted Publications.

Orr, K., and R. Simmons. 2010. "Dual Identities: The In-service Teacher Trainee Experience in the English Further Education Sector." *Journal of Vocational Education & Training* 62 (1): 75–88.

Ranson, S. 2003. "Public Accountability in the Age of Neo-liberal Governance." *Journal of Education Policy* 18 (5): 459–480.

Rustin, M. 2013. "A Relational Society." In *After Neoliberalism? A Kilburn Manifesto*, edited by S. Hall, D. Massey, and M. Rustin. Soundings: A Journal of Politics and Culture. Accessed August 2, 2014. http://www.lwbooks.co.uk/journals/soundings/pdfs/Soundings%20Manifesto_Rustin.pdf

Salisbury, J., M. Jephcote, G. Rees, and J. Roberts. 2006. "Emotional Labour, Ethics of Care: Work Intensification in FE Colleges." Working paper presented at British Educational Research Association Annual Conference, University of Warwick, September 6–9. Accessed January 15, 2014. http://www.furthereducationresearch.org/working.htm

Sedgmore, L. 2014. "'Dear Minister' – an Open Letter to Nick Boles." FE Opinion, *Times Education Supplement*. Accessed August 11, 2014. https://news.tes.co.uk/further-education/b/opinion/2014/08/06/39-dear-minister-39-an-open-letter-to-nick-boles.aspx

Shore, S., and E. Butler. 2012. "Missing Things and Methodological Swerves: Unsettling the It-ness of VET." *International Journal of Training Research* 10 (3): 204–218.

Simmons, R. 2008. "Gender, Work and Identity: A Case Study from the English Further Education Sector." *Research in Post-Compulsory Education* 13 (3): 267–279.

Skills Commission. 2010. *Teacher Training in Vocational Education. Skills Policy Connect*. London: Edge Foundation.

Smith, R., and M. O'Leary. 2013. "NPM in an Age of Austerity: Knowledge and Experience in Further Education." *Journal of Educational Administration and History* 45 (3): 244–266.

Teaching and Learning Research Programme and Economic and Social Research Council (TLRP and ESRC). 2008. *Challenges and Change in Further Education*. London: Institute of Education.

Tipton, B. 1973. *Conflict and Change in a Technical College*. Hutchinson: Brunel University Monographs.

University and College Union (UCU). 2013. "Developing a National Framework for the Effective Use of Lesson Observation in Further Education." Project Report. Accessed November 2013. http://www.ucu.org.uk/7105

Venables, E. 1968. *The Young Worker at College. A Study of a Local Tech*. London: Faber and Faber.

Wragg, E. C. 1999. *An Introduction to Classroom Observation*. 2nd ed. London: Routledge.

The impact of lecturers' initial teacher training on continuing professional development needs for teaching and learning in post-compulsory education

Gary Husband

This paper presents the initial findings of a research project that aims to investigate the impact of teacher training for lecturers in post-compulsory education on engagement with continuing professional development (CPD) for learning and teaching. The majority of colleges and universities operating in the UK now ensure that all teaching staff are given access to training in skills for learning and teaching. This training can take many different forms and this paper explores the potential differences in outcome and influence on engagement with CPD and lifelong learning of graduates from these programmes. For the study, 18 lecturers from different colleges (one large multi-campus college in Scotland and another in Wales) provided narrative accounts about their professional background, training and qualifications prior to initial lecturer training and their route into teaching in further education. Respondents then engaged in semi-structured interviews about their experiences in lecturer training and ongoing engagement with CPD and further learning post-training. The findings indicate that respondents feel insufficient emphasis is placed on vocational skills training, meeting special educational needs and classroom management techniques. Lecturers agree that CPD in learning and teaching is very important but the research data show lack of meaningful engagement with the training options currently available. Recommendations are made to colleges to increase the practical and vocational focus and content of teacher training for lecturers whilst acknowledging the importance of allowing novice practitioner status. The requirement for access to high-quality, valid and targeted CPD is highlighted, with lecturers acknowledging the importance of training and expressing the desire to engage with relevant courses in learning and teaching.

Introduction

This research aims to investigate the impact of initial teacher training for lecturers in post-compulsory education on engagement with continuing professional development (CPD) for learning and teaching by:

(1) evaluating the efficacy of models of initial teacher training in post-compulsory education by identifying any skills or knowledge deficiencies as described by respondent lecturers, and

(2) analysing the effects of initial teacher training for lecturers in post-compulsory education on individuals' attitudes and approach towards CPD and further qualifications in the field of learning and teaching.

The needs of students studying in further and higher education institutions are diverse and often complex in nature (Lea and Callaghan 2006). The facilitation of student learning by lecturers in post-compulsory education requires a high level of skill and deep understanding of the theory and practices of learning and teaching. Initial lecturer training in these sectors takes many forms and varies in length, depth and quality of provision (Skills Commission 2010). A programme of CPD under-taken by lecturers is widely regarded in the post-compulsory education sector as an important part of professional practice. As the needs of students accessing education and training in both sectors change and develop, there is a compelling argument that lecturers also need to update skills, engage with changing theories of education and share good practice, an enhancement of the sector through professional development (Evans 2008). The university and college sectors for many years fulfilled different roles in society but these defined functions are now becoming blurred as commonalities, articulation and partnerships become more prevalent.

Expectations of the teaching and learning experience have changed in all areas of post-compulsory education as students are encouraged to take a role in the leader-ship and development of institutions through student associations. Students in many ways view themselves as customers and this is having an impact on acceptance of the quality of teaching and resources.

A case study carried out by the researcher (Husband 2012) indicated that there was a link between initial lecturer training and ongoing engagement with CPD in learning and teaching. In semi-structured interviews, respondents (all qualified lec-turers) recounted their experiences of initial teacher training and discussed the areas in which they felt they needed further training and development. The case study highlighted potential problems with the training provided for lecturers in some FE colleges that influenced lecturers' ongoing engagement with lifelong learning and professional development. This study builds on that work and further investigates some of the issues raised.

There is a large body of work and research published surrounding the issues of content of initial lecturer training courses (Avis et al. 2012; Brandon and Charlton 2011; Lucas and Unwin 2009), but little on the impact on engagement with CPD and continued education in teaching and learning. This research aims to add to that body of work by exploring in greater depth the influence of lecturer training on individuals who undertake it and identifying any perceived gaps in training provision.

This research utilises narrative accounts (Yin 2011) and semi-structured inter-views (Dawson 2009; Mason 2002) to ascertain which predominant influences on lecturers have the greatest impact on the practices of teaching and learning. The foreground issues are related to the models of training in further education (FE) and academic staff development in higher education (HE) that are predominant in current practice.

This paper discusses the commonalities between teaching and learning practices in HE and FE and the implications these may have for future training of lecturers. Commonly used models of lecturer training in use in both HE and FE are explored and analysed. The paper goes on to report the findings of the research after completing a total of 18 interviews in March and April of 2014 with lecturers from two separate further education colleges, one large multi-campus college in Scotland and another in Wales.

FE and HE

Structure and curriculum

The ways in which universities and colleges function within society have traditionally been perceived as very different by students, industry stakeholders and academic communities. Further education colleges have traditionally provided opportunities to learn a vocation, support communities and empower individuals to achieve their economic goals (Nwabude and Ade-Ojo 2008). Universities have traditionally provided a more academic route into areas such as history, pure mathematics, philosophy and literature, with higher-skilled vocations such as medicine and veterinary science also forming large parts of curricula. Universities have always been independent of a national curriculum or prescription in delivery but have benefitted from public funding, enabling them to research and teach independently with minimum government influence and restriction (Boulton and Lucas 2008). Universities have different focuses and do not all follow the same curriculum, systems and delivery methods. Pre-1992 (Further and Higher Education Act 1992) universities, including the Russell Group universities, may have a greater focus on securing funding from various sources for research, whereas post-1992 universities are more likely to focus heavily on the teaching of students. All universities are different in nature and as such have unique ethos, focus and staff, and the approaches to CPD and training for teaching and learning are as diverse as the sector itself. Colleges have always been influenced heavily by government strategy and the industrial needs of the country but each has its own distinguishing features.

Some colleges have a focus on state-funded full-time education, others may specialise in apprenticeship schemes and privately funded training. Colleges have been perceived as a source for training in skilled manual labour and an environment in which individuals pursuing vocational training, adult learning or community support programmes can flourish (Simmons 2008).

These different influences brought about different development and cultures within the two sectors, however these boundaries are now blurring, especially in the post-1992 universities, some of which developed from FE colleges (Burkill, Dyer, and Stone 2008; Feather 2012; Gallacher 2006).

The academic culture within further education colleges has developed to be very similar to that in schools (Simmons 2008). Until 1992, all colleges came under the jurisdiction and control of the local education authorities that manage and run schools. The Further and Higher Education Act of 1992 (Government UK 1992) set up colleges as corporations that directly employed their own staff. Colleges continue to offer highly structured courses developed in conjunction with industry, delivered in a scaffolded programme complementing apprenticeships (latterly, modern apprenticeship frameworks) and working life.

In contrast to this, many universities have developed highly specialised research departments, programmes, projects and staff, and are ideally placed to immerse students, both undergraduate and postgraduate, in a complete learning experience through lectures and engagement with research for advancement of knowledge, policy and teaching (Wend 2013).

Teaching and learning

The methods and processes of teaching in universities have not until recent years undergone any national scrutiny in terms of formalisation, standardisation and quality control. The Dearing Report in 1997 began the process of scrutinising learning and teaching in universities. The Economic and Social Research Council, funded by the Higher Education Funding Council for England, began a project in 2000 to review the quality of teaching and learning across the entire education system.

Ensuring quality of provision for the range and ability of individuals accessing post-compulsory education presents a variety of challenges to institutions (Orr 2010). A lecturer in an FE college can now be presented with a group of 14-year-olds accessing basic vocational training, 16–60-year-olds accessing a range of courses and students undertaking HE modules and degrees. Each represented group has its own needs and requirements, which will vary widely – one set of skills or standards may not be sufficient in ensuring parity in quality of provision across the whole post-compulsory education sector.

In many instances the traditional role of universities as research establishments remains and, for a significant proportion, individual institutions' international recognition and reputation are based on this output (Parsons et al. 2012). However, the Organisation for Economic Cooperation and Development has completed pilot studies in measuring and comparing student ability on leaving university and is now considering rolling out 'The Assessment of Higher Education Learning Outcomes' project internationally (Mathews 2013). This in itself is in response to the changing attitudes of students towards universities and the focus of communities accessing education and training.

The increase in tuition fees payable by students and the introduction of university league tables have given rise to greater expectations of quality from students now accessing provision as customers (Svensson and Wood 2007). Students are encouraged to scrutinise overall experience, quality of provision, perceived lecturer standards and resources, whilst student associations now play a greater role in the running and management of organisations.

Expectations of direct classroom delivery, smaller tuition groups and increased tutor support are more akin to traditional school teaching, perhaps especially that of sixth-form provision, and are in contrast to the traditional view of subject immersion, assimilation and self-discovery. University league tables (Times Higher Education, Reuters, The Complete University Guide) ranking institutions on the number of teaching-qualified lecturing staff, successful completion statistics and resources are now being used by students to assess the perceived quality of provision and value for money offered by different universities across the UK and world. Students now increasingly expect a higher level of attention and individual service – it does not necessarily follow that this provides a greater quality of teaching but it does change the required approach to learning and teaching by lecturers.

This change in stance presents challenges for many working in universities in terms of professional identity – are they lecturers that research or researchers that teach (Alruz and Khasawneh 2013; Clegg 2012; Drennan, Clark, and Hyde 2013)? The professional identity of practitioners within universities could be a major influencing factor on engagement with learning and teaching skills and practice. This is, of course, highly individualistic in nature: academic background, personal beliefs and institutional culture all having significant influence (Whitchurch 2008).

Universities are responding in a variety of ways, for instance mandatory teacher training specific to higher education for new lecturers and pay awards for existing staff that undertake training and professional recognition from the Higher Education Academy. These changes in practice now reflect the established stance in FE and underline the increased importance being placed on training for teaching and learning.

However, there is a fear that over prescription in teaching methods, focus on league tables for teaching and learning and international quality assessment will homogenise higher education and in many ways make it mirror the standard school system (Lueger and Vettori 2008). The possibility that prescriptive curriculum and delivery will lead to outcome-based, standardised assessment is very real, as has happened in FE.

CPD

The pre- and post-devolution landscape of the UK has presented many different versions of professional standards for lecturers and trainers in colleges. Regionalised and overarching standards have formed the basis for practice, training and CPD for many years.

The UK Professional Standards Framework (UKPSF) for teaching and supporting learning in HE (HEA 2011) is the current set of descriptors endorsed by the Higher Education Academy for use in universities. As lecturers develop and demonstrate the core values and skills, they are awarded increased professional status and recognition.

Scrutiny of the standards for FE (New Overarching Standards, England, Northern Ireland, Scotland and Wales) and the UKPSF suggests that they have similar focus, structure and intention, yet there is no crossover between qualifications; FE- and HE-specific training does not allow for a crossover into working in both sectors and separate qualifications are often mandatory.

The time frame in which lecturer training takes place and the various formats followed do not allow for all eventualities and specialisms to be covered. Lecturers, throughout their careers, will constantly be exposed to new experiences and ideas that will form the basis of ongoing professional skill development that complements and informs the requirements for CPD. Specialist subject areas such as student support for special educational needs (SEN) (medical, social and emotional, see Spenceley [2012]) or managing challenging behaviour are continually developing as societal needs change and awareness of SEN becomes more of a focus in FE. Time for lecturers to engage in a programme of CPD is challenging to find in ever increasingly financially constrained organisations, where lecturers are operating in more stringently timetabled regimes. The financial constraints imposed over the last five years are also placing extreme pressure on the funding for the delivery of training and colleges are turning to their own staff to provide in-house training for peers. Nearly all colleges now offer a programme of CPD available to teaching staff, and this research looks at engagement with and uptake of the courses and sessions available.

Models of lecturer training

There are various different ways in which training to teach in both FE and universities is undertaken. Many training courses are undertaken by teachers whilst they are fulfilling contracts and managing a full timetable of teaching and/or research. Some trainees are given a remission in teaching obligation to undertake studies, but many are not (Lucas and Unwin 2009).

Further education colleges access external provision from universities for many courses as the level of teaching qualification is often at undergraduate or postgraduate level and requires the validation of the higher education establishment providing the training.

This provision can be delivered using several different methods:

(1) delivered at the university full- or part-time
(2) in-house at the college delivered under licence by college staff
(3) in-house at the college delivered by university staff
(4) distance learning via university online provision
(5) blended mixture of distance learning and classroom tuition (both in-house and external).

The majority of teaching courses require the learner to be observed in a teaching role in their normal place of work.

The depth and scope of the training courses vary depending on geographical location, teaching contract and institution type. In Scotland, only full-time lecturers have to undertake the Teaching Qualification in Further Education (TQ[FE]: Postgraduate Certificate in Education, FE equivalent) training, which can only be done at one of three providing universities: Aberdeen, Dundee and Stirling. However, the depth and scope of the Scottish TQ(FE) are truncated in comparison to the English/ Welsh model (Avis et al. 2012). In England, Wales and Northern Ireland, the current legislation is under review (Independent Review Panel 2012) to ascertain the best way to develop the sector but the traditional model utilised in recent years has been a part-time, two-year programme containing 120 credits at level 6/7.

Universities will access many similar provisions but where possible will utilise and develop their own in-house validated provision. The courses are generally modular in nature, taught at postgraduate level, vary between classroom delivery, online and blended learning and are accredited by the Higher Education Academy. Undoubtedly there are advantages to all models.

Online, blended and social learning environments

The utilisation of online learning gives freedom of access to resources, removes time constraints imposed by attendance models and allows for opportunity to access a wider social group of trainees through online blogs, social media interaction and course-specific forums. Communities of practice engaging with online learning may come from a wider expertise base, greater geographical area and extended subject specialisms, all providing greater diversity and potentially depth to the trainee's experience (Khoo, Forret, and Cowie 2009; Wenger 1998).

Whilst online learning provides opportunities for flexibility, traditional classroom delivery also has many advantages. Individuals engaged in training meet regularly and engage in discussion, practical demonstration, vocational participation and can engage in an expansive learning environment (Lucas and Unwin 2009). Teaching can be more structured and assurance of immersion in subject matter can be more easily guaranteed, that is, trainees are routinely exposed to all theories and ideas presented in class, whereas online learning may allow for a trainee to skip sections deemed important (Orvis et al. 2010), struggle with meaning or feel isolated in their learning (Centre for Applied Research 2003). The culture of the institution instigating the training programme is a crucial influencing factor on the engagement with and scope of learning of its trainees – expansive and restrictive approaches yielding differing results and methods (O'Leary 2013). Research in this area suggests that there are several benefits to providing students with inclusive social models of training (Boyd, Allan, and Reale 2010; Wenger 1998). In an environment where trainees are routinely involved with peers on a regular basis, opportunities arise for sharing of experience and open acknowledgement of novice status whilst maintaining legitimate professional participation within their academic departments. This allows for regular reflection and review and enables trainees to experiment with ideas, compare experiences and form professional relationships (Harkin, Clow, and Hillier 2003; Scottish Government 2012) – a safe environment in which to practise and become competent without negative impact. The vocational nature of teaching is reflected in this practical method of teaching and developing competence.

The development of learning groups in training situations in many ways reflects the formation of a community of practice, in this instance a community of novice practitioners.

Lave and Wenger (2002, 115) describe a community of practice as:

> ... participation in an activity system about which participants share understandings concerning what they are doing and what that means in their lives and for their communities.

This can be applied to a learning community in which trainees and newly qualified teaching staff are developing their participation and skill levels. A community of practice should be centred on the development of trainees and continued research into new and best practice for training teachers in FE and HE, with inclusive participation of the trainees themselves.

A community of practice does not have to exist solely within an organisation, but can be accessed by the wider community, across sectors and institutions. Some trainees have benefitted from access to an online learning community that reinforced the taught sessions, provided support for trainees whilst at work or on placement and gave access to important information and interactive training resources (Hramiak 2010; Khoo, Forret, and Cowie 2009). The forming of communities of practice that offer support for individuals and allow the sharing of best practice can be aided by online enhancement for learning. Many establishments involved in training have started to utilise a blended learning approach. Utilisation of online written resources, webinars and virtual learning environments, coupled with some classroom and vocational contact as a method of providing training, can offer enhanced learning opportunities but the reduction in vocational training time offers some challenges to teacher educators (Holley and Oliver 2010). However, embracing a blended learning strategy, using elements of both classroom taught sessions and online delivery, can ensure that trainees are exposed to the better parts of both online and classroom delivery models (Hughes 2007).

This method can allow trainees to form wider social circles and utilise a more diverse skill set learned in both practical and online scenarios. The increasing levels of usability in technology available in virtual learning environment support and blended learning are enabling academic staff to create innovative and engaging learning tools for students (Ashraf 2009). Online learning is moving on from being a repository for information and evolving into an interactive environment for learning (Laurillard 2008).

Mentors

The approach to training of institutions, whether it be in-house, external, online or blended, may have an effect on the engagement with training of individuals. The importance placed upon lecturer training by an institution, including provision for mentor support and remission, in time may also have an effect on student engagement and motivation.

Much has been written regarding the importance and models of mentor support for student teachers (Gay 1994; Ingleby 2011; Mutton, Mills, and McNicholl 2006; Scandura et al. 1996; Valenčič and Vogrinc 2007; Woodd 1997). Although the researcher acknowledges the effect of mentors in a developmental role, no specific emphasis is placed on extending the research in this field as part of this study. However, the pastoral role of a mentor within a structured collegial programme may prove to have an effect on trainees' engagement with their current and future training (Cunningham 2007).

The role of the mentor is afforded varying importance in different institutions in both FE and HE. Some institutions ensure that each trainee is matched with a suitable mentor (for experience and specialist skills) and both trainee and mentor follow an agreed programme until the period of training is finished. Some institutions place less significance on the role of the mentor, and a 'peer pal' system (Woodd 1997) is utilised to aid the trainee. The nature of this study may elicit information regarding these relationships that could provide interesting insights into individual motivation and the strengths and weaknesses of mentor relationships.

Research approach

The research utilised semi-structured interviews with individual lecturers (Dawson 2009; Mason 2002). The data were taken directly from the teaching professionals as the focus of the project relates specifically to training, experiences and opinions of the lecturing staff it is investigating. Direct interaction with the lecturers enables the researcher to reveal the effects of training models and sector practices on the unique journey of individuals to qualified lecturer status. The lecturers are able to reflect on their own feelings and opinions on teaching-related CPD and the perception of their professional identity.

The lecturers are encouraged to produce a narrative account recalling their own learning journey. Narrative research methods (i.e., recounting verbally, personal learning experiences and giving account of feelings and ideas) have been used widely in educational research (Thody 2006; Wertz and Charmaz 2011). In this research, utilisation of narrative methods in the initial stages of the interview enabled the respondent lecturer to contextualise their position and respond openly and frankly regarding agency and identity. Utilising individuals' narrative accounts allows the researcher to perform phenomenological analysis and gain an understanding of the importance to respondents of circumstance and experience (Andrews, Squire, and Tamboukou 2008). Encouraging the respondent to relate his or her own story gives rise to descriptive opportunity that can yield information that may not have been forthcoming using a questionnaire approach. In this research, this method was found to be useful as all of the respondents have very different backgrounds, training and professional specialisms.

Although the face-to-face interaction with individual respondents took place in one session, two methods for the gathering of data were employed. The continuation of the conversation in the form of a semi-structured interview afforded the interviewer the opportunity to explore areas of interest that arose from the narrative (Yin 2011). Semi-structured interviews are widely used in education research (Drever 2003) to enable respondents to give descriptive accounts and relate experience to direct questions. This method helps ensure that the researcher is able to maintain a level of control over the direction of the interview but allows for respondent freedom of expression that otherwise may be stifled.

The research project aims to seek input from teacher-qualified lecturers in both colleges of further education and universities (pre- and post-92). Two colleges of further education and two universities were selected for geographical location, size of establishment and similarities in operating model, one in Scotland and the other Wales; the researcher has experience of working in both these areas of the UK. Initial approaches were made via named contacts and permission to approach staff was sought and received. Named contacts agreed to circulate information regarding the research to colleagues and respondents were contacted directly by the researcher. All British Educational Research Association guidelines and ethical rules were followed closely and the respondents were given full information pertinent to all aspects of the project prior to involvement (BERA 2011). The research received ethical approval from the appropriate ethics committee at Bangor University.

Respondents were sought within organisations without focus on their subject specialisms. Teacher educators have not been included at this stage as this phase of the research aims to focus on the responses of specialists whose focus is the students of the organisation and not staff development. The interviews took approximately 40 minutes with the first 5–10 minutes being devoted to narrative from respondents.

The initial scope of this project was to carry out a comparative study that encompassed responses from practitioners working in all areas of post-compulsory education. The included review of literature gives a detailed and important overview of the policies, issues and developing commonalities across a wide cross-section of post-compulsory education. Two sectors (FE and HE), traditionally distinctly viewed, have been shown to have several areas of commonality. As the project has progressed, both circumstance and scale have become important factors for consideration. This paper focuses on the responses from a first round of interviews with lecturers working in FE and offers insight and analysis into the thoughts and perceptions exclusively of teaching practitioners in this sector. Reporting on the findings at this stage presents an important opportunity to explore the headline issues as reported by lecturers. Results and recommendations informing practices specific to FE are included that could inform the design and implementation of development programmes and policy in colleges, enabling training to meet the professional needs identified by the practitioners themselves.

Moving forward, the second phase of this research will be concerned with conducting follow-up interviews focused specifically at exploring further the headline issues presented in this paper. The second phase of interviews will include responses from teacher educators/trainers, policy makers and college managers, giving the research increased scope and depth and an alternative perspective.

Requests made at the outset of this project to selected universities yielded permission to make interview requests of lecturers. Time constraints and professional obligations of university lecturers at the time of approach may have accounted for the poor response to the request for respondents, however, this situation has presented an opportunity to increase the depth of analysis and scope of this project. A similar project looking at the same issues is being conducted by an experienced researcher working in one of the approached universities who has focused exclusively on the responses of lecturers in this sector. A proposed partnership will yield the third phase of this research and produce a paper reporting on the issues commonly affecting lecturers in both sectors. An ongoing collaboration may yield further opportunities for development and improvement in the training provided to lecturers across post-compulsory education and the sharing of best practice through an articulated approach.

Data analysis

As the research process continued and more interviews were completed, each set of generated data was reviewed using inductive thematic analysis. A total of 18 interviews were conducted generating over 11 hours of raw data. Questions were digitally grouped using Livescribe software and reviewed in numerical order as groups, for example all responses to Q1 together.

Common responses were identified and logged on a chart, which was then analysed for emergent themes. These themes were further explored in subsequent interviews with respondents from similar backgrounds. The research evolved to explore in greater depth issues repeatedly raised by lecturers and ensure that a point of data saturation was reached. Themes and commonality were identified and coded to ensure that the data-set was thoroughly examined for recurring phenomena and information that was pertinent to the specific area of study (Davies 2007). Comparative analysis helped mitigate the problem of working with a large data-set; all coded responses were grouped and analysed together to look for commonalities in the answers or recurrent phenomena in the wider data-set (Andrews, Squire, and Tamboukou 2008).

Findings and emergent themes

These findings are taken from interviews carried out up to May 2014. Emergent themes are becoming evident and further investigation is required for future publication. A second round of interviews with lecturers in FE is being conducted utilising the same methods but incorporating further questions to further explore the findings outlined below. The second round of interviews will include responses from lecturer trainers/educators, policy makers and educational managers.

The initial hypothesis for this research was concerned with the impact of differing models on engagement with CPD in learning and teaching. A small-scale case study (Husband 2012) appeared to indicate that graduates from dissimilar models of training showed differing propensities to continue with any form of CPD. At present, the findings of the initial case study are not being corroborated by this research. There does not appear to be a link in overall engagement with any form of CPD from dissimilar models of training but the data suggest that there is a link between type and model of training and specific CPD needs.

Narrative accounts

Analysis of the narrative accounts given by respondents gave a very clear picture of the type of people practising teaching in FE. The narratives varied in length and depth but all respondents recounted the professional journey that they had taken to lead them into a career in FE. Most were university graduates, with many having completed their degrees and higher degrees later in their careers. All had worked previously within the industry in which they were experts or had significant professional experience to enable competent delivery across subject areas, for example health and safety, core/essential skills and maths in engineering. Those who did not hold university degrees were professional graduates who had completed apprenticeships and had gone on to complete higher levels of study such as Higher National Certificate/Diploma (HNC/D).

Only individuals who had undertaken teacher training for secondary school practice had undertaken any form of training prior to commencement of employment within FE. All were fully qualified with a range of graduate/postgraduate courses completed including, Postgraduate Certificate in Education (PGCE), Professional Graduate Diploma in Education (PGDE), PGCE(FE) and TQ(FE). All respondents with PGCE(FE) and TQ(FE) had undertaken this training whilst working as lecturers in an FE context. All reported having enjoyed large parts of their training and felt it had overall been of benefit and a positive experience. For many it was a departure from what had previously been entirely technical training and it was an opportunity to develop wider academic skills. Many reported making lasting friendships during training and most still enjoyed good professional relations formed during training courses.

Vocational pedagogy

A significant part of the vocational skill in learning and teaching is demonstrated in the ability to effectively manage a learning environment, meet SEN and overcome challenging behaviour, whilst ensuring that students are valued as individuals and are given the space in which to develop. Many respondents felt that their training had partially covered this area but had not prepared them sufficiently to manage this crucial aspect of their role. A female lecturer practising in Wales who now undertakes the responsibility to mentor some trainee lecturers made the following observation:

> As a mentor I walk into [trainee and newly qualified lecturers'] classrooms and often find total chaos and the lecturer does not know how to deal with it or stop it happening, they have not been taught this.

This identified the possibility of skills and knowledge deficiency in trainee and newly qualified lecturers. This was discussed by many of the respondents who reflected on the difficulties they faced in the early stages of their careers. A female lecturer practising in Wales gave the following reflection:

> Of the two years training I did, the first year was the most useful, I was struggling with some students and classes and the stuff they taught helped me get through, it was good, I wanted more at the time.

In the interviews a large proportion of respondents identified they felt they needed to seek specific further training in classroom management and meeting SEN as this had not been covered satisfactorily in initial training. The only people who did not identify this were the respondents who had completed PGCE/PGDE training in secondary schools but are now working in FE.

A male lecturer practising in Wales commented:

> I feel there was very little on how to handle students, difficult students or students that were emotional or had certain difficulties. These skills were learned on the job after the course. In some respects the training did not get us classroom ready.

A male lecturer practising in Scotland stated:

> If I'm being really blunt, I found that the qualification didn't make me a better teacher. I didn't find that it gave me anything practical that I would then take away and use in class the next day, I found that odd.

These sentiments were reflected on by a large proportion of respondents who all felt that practical pedagogy had been missed from the curriculum, or 'glossed over' as a female lecturer from Scotland phrased it, and who went on to say:

> There was little in the way of tangible practical training and the lecturer [after an observed assessed session] was more concerned that I had missed an opportunity to embed core skills but could offer no real advice on how to deal with the disruption in the class.

All respondents who had undertaken a TQ(FE) in Scotland identified lack of practical training in their course as an issue that they had tried to address with in-house and external training post-qualification with limited success. All interviewed graduates of FE-specific courses identified the importance of the practical aspects of their training yet none were fully satisfied, irrespective of model, with the experience and support for classroom management available during training. Many respondents felt that their subject specialism knowledge was up to and beyond the required standard but often felt that poor skills in classroom management hindered their performance as effective lecturers. A large proportion identified, when asked, that in their opinion the primary function of lecturer training should be vocational teaching skills training. Several respondents made comments such as this from a male lecturer from Wales:

> You need to learn the skills to put it over [subject matter] and you need the tools to do this well.

A female lecturer from Wales said:

> You need to learn the skills to manage and plan and develop the tool kit to help you in the classroom and to operate successfully.

A male lecturer from Scotland responded:

> People come from different backgrounds and it's really important that they are taught the skills needed to teach and manage students.

This demonstrates awareness amongst lecturers of the importance of training but also highlights their desires and what they feel should be the primary focus of the training provided.

All respondents identified the practical aspects of their training as most valuable and useful in subsequent teaching practice. Micro-teaching strategies in PGCE(FE) and placements in PGCE/PGDE were identified as providing safe spaces in which to practise and become proficient in many teaching skills.

One of several similar comments from respondents came from a female lecturer in Wales:

> In the early stages of training I found the micro-teaching sessions to be most useful. Although nerve wracking, the sessions taught us how to structure and deliver a formative session.

The use of micro-teaching was commented upon favourably as it gave individuals a safe space in which to try out ideas, deliver a session where mistakes had no detriment and peer review provided a positive platform for support and development.

The distance learning mode of delivery on a part-time basis was identified as being problematic but the consensus amongst respondents was that they believed the universities providing the training were in a difficult position. Colleges are increasingly reducing the time given to trainees; in fact, many had received no time from their employer in which to train, and all study had been undertaken whilst completing the full timetable and responsibilities of a lecturer. A female lecturer in Scotland reflected positively on her overall training quality and experience but made the following observation:

> The gradual increase in training over three years worked really well but as I became more experienced my work responsibilities increased as did the demands of the training course. The expectation to train over and above a full-time job was very challenging in the end.

CPD

All respondents agreed that CPD was vital to the ongoing development and professional conduct of lecturers but very few actively engaged in CPD in the area that they highlighted as needing most development – SEN and classroom management. However, one respondent male lecturer from Wales made the following observation:

> I don't have time for CPD. I'm contracted to deliver 800 hours of teaching in a year, I am currently up to 860 hours. I would love to go and do X, Y and Z but I can't because I simply do not have the time.

This highlights the potential problems in delivering CPD in FE. Time constraints, subject specialists and available materials are all possible contributing factors. Of greater concern may be the possibility that the sector does not have an understanding of the deficit in training as identified by staff.

Some respondents were quite scathing of CPD programmes available to them within their organisations. A female lecturer in Scotland commented:

> We get very little time for CPD, when we do want to go to something we can't get classes covered and then we are expected to go to stuff that is either not relevant or poorly prepared. It is really hard to find really good training that answers questions and gives good ideas.

Many felt that the provision of CPD was piecemeal and only available to fulfil external audit requirements. The majority of respondents identified that they had done no meaningful CPD in teaching and learning post-teacher training. This amounts to a very low uptake in CPD for teaching and learning for lecturers, which is interesting when most respondents stated that CPD was vital to a lecturer and the ongoing development of the sector. A lecturer practising in Wales made the following comment:

> I have done all the mandatory training expected of me over the last few years but I don't see that as CPD, I got little from it. I have done a lot of other courses that I elected to study and these have proved to be really important and now I feel I can give a richer learner experience.

This raises questions over the quality of mandatory training, availability of relevant courses and accessibility of high-quality further developmental training in teaching and learning. Most respondents were fully engaged in subject specialism CPD and many respondents had completed, were starting or are halfway through higher degrees in subject specialist areas.

Concluding remarks and possibilities for further research

This research has shown that lecturers in FE are acutely aware of the need for training, the continued necessity for engagement with CPD and the professional requirement to continually maintain and develop skills. The desire to undertake high-quality CPD in subjects and areas of concern and interest to lecturers is palpable but many barriers were highlighted. Lack of availability, quality of provision, relevance of subject matter and workload are all causes of concern that colleges should take seriously.

The research has shown that initial lecturer training is a positive experience but it is leaving lecturers feeling that they have a skills shortage in important areas. Many respondents commented on the good quality of teaching surrounding the management of curriculum and the structures within FE; all felt prepared and able to practise proficiently within the sector having graduated from training. Many lecturers were struggling with fundamental skills essential to proactive classroom management and many made suggestions that they were not afforded the right to practise at a novice level prior to full engagement with all responsibilities of the role of a lecturer, despite in many cases being remunerated at a novice rate. The removal of time to train within work and the lack of acknowledgement of novice status were highlighted as challenges and possible causes of stress amongst trainee lecturers.

The universities providing the TQ(FE) provision in Scotland are having to facilitate the learning of trainee lecturers in truncated timescales and increasingly few personal contact opportunities. The expectations of many trainee lecturers are now not being fully met.

Colleges may need to address the vocational pedagogical skills training prior to attendance on TQ(FE) with supplementary courses such as Professional Development Awards delivered in-house.

Many areas of learning must be covered in lecturer training and sufficient academic standard achieved by all individuals to graduate at (often) postgraduate level. Is it feasible to place a greater emphasis on the vocational skills of teaching within modern initial lecturer training within the limited time constraints? How would courses that utilise a largely distance learning model incorporate greater skills training in classroom management and meeting SEN?

There is a distinct possibility that effective classroom management skills are only developed over an extended time period and have a direct positive correlation with experience and exposure to high-risk and vulnerable groups. Is it therefore possible to fully train individual lecturers in the short initial training period to deal with all possible eventualities and to be confident in their abilities?

Limitations of this research

Using narrative and semi-skilled interview methods is time consuming and requires considerable organisation. The research has a projected timescale of two years from start to completion.

Utilising narrative and semi-structured interviews generates a very large amount of information and data. It is expected that up to 30 respondents may need to be interviewed in this project to ensure that a wide range of issues are covered and data saturation is achieved (Saldana 2011). Utilisation of coding to identify themes ensured that all responses were scrutinised thoroughly for meaning and inference. All coded statements were placed in a matrix to cross-reference responses from individual respondents and ensure that thematic interpretation of commonly occurring statements was consistent. The qualitative nature of the information could lead to problems of misinterpretation and the possibility of researcher bias. Peer review (whilst maintaining all ethical considerations of anonymity and privacy) of all data interpretation was carried out and all conclusions drawn from data were scrutinised by an independent third party to ensure that no bias was being introduced by the researcher/author.

Acknowledgements
The author would like to acknowledge the support of Dr Charles Buckley and Dr David Sullivan.

Disclosure statement
No potential conflict of interest was reported by the author.

References
Alruz, J., and S. Khasawneh. 2013. "Professional Identity of Faculty Members at Higher Education Institutions: A Criterion for Workplace Success." *Research in Post-Compulsory Education* 18 (4): 431–442.

Andrews, M., C. Squire, and M. Tamboukou. 2008. *Doing Narrative Research*. London: Sage.

Ashraf, B. 2009. "Teaching the Google-eyed YouTube Generation." *Journal of Education and Training* 51 (5–6): 343–352.

Avis, J., R. Canning, R. Fisher, B. Morgan-Klein, and R. Simmons. 2012. "State Intervention and Teacher Education for Vocational Educators in England and Scotland." *Journal of Educational Research* 54 (2): 187–197.

Boulton, G., and C. Lucas. 2008. *What Are Universities for?* Leuven, Belgium: League of European Research Universities.

Boyd, P., S. Allan, and P. Reale. 2010. "Being a Teacher Educator: Pedagogy, Scholarship and Identity of Lecturers in Teacher Education in Further Education Workplace Contexts." University of Cumbria. Accessed July 15. 2012. http://www.cumbria.ac.uk/Public/Education/Documents/Research/EducatorsStorehouse/TeachereducatorsinFEColleges.pdf

Brandon, T., and J. Charlton. 2011. "The Lessons Learned from Developing an Inclusive Learning and Teaching Community of Practice." *International Journal of Inclusive Education* 15 (1): 165–178.

British Educational Research Association. 2011. *Ethical Guidelines for Educational Research.* London: Author.

Burkill, S., S. Dyer, and M. Stone. 2008. "Lecturing in Higher Education in Further Education Settings." *Journal of Further and Higher Education* 32 (4): 321–331.

Centre for Applied Research. 2003. "Impact and Challenges of E Learning." In *Supporting E Learning in Higher Education*, Vol. 3, 39–47. Accessed March 15, 2013. https://net.edu cause.edu/ir/library/pdf/ers0303/rs/ers03036.pdf

Clegg, S. 2012. "Conceptualising Higher Education Research and/or Academic Development as 'Fields': A Critical Analysis." *Higher Education Research & Development* 31 (5): 667–678.

Cunningham, B. 2007. "All the Right Features: Towards an 'Architecture' for Mentoring Trainee Teachers in UK Further Education Colleges." *Journal of Education for Teaching* 33 (1): 83–97.

Davies, M. 2007. *Doing a Successful Research Project.* London: Palgrave Macmillan.

Dawson, C. 2009. *Introduction to Research Methods: A Practical Guide for Anyone Undertaking a Research Project.* London: How To Books.

Drennan, J., M. Clark, and A. Hyde. 2013. "Professional Identity in Higher Education." In *The Academic Profession in Europe: New Tasks and New Challenges*, edited by B. Kehm and U. Teichler, 7–21. London: Springer.

Drever, E. 2003. *Using Semi Structured Interviews in Small Scale Research.* 2nd ed. Glasgow: The SCRE Centre, University of Glasgow.

Evans, L. 2008. "Professionalism, Professionality and the Development of Education." *British Journal of Educational Studies* 56 (1): 20–38.

Feather, D. 2012. "Oh to Be a Scholar: An HE in FE Perspective." *Journal of Further and Higher Education* 36 (2): 243–261.

Gallacher, J. 2006. "Blurring the Boundaries or Creating Diversity? The Contribution of the Further Education Colleges to Higher Education in Scotland." *Journal of Further and Higher Education* 30 (1): 43–58.

Gay, B. 1994. "What is Mentoring?" *Journal of Education and Training* 36 (5): 4–7.

Harkin, J., R. Clow, and Y. Hillier. 2003. "Recollected in Tranquillity? FE Teachers' Perceptions of Their Initial Teacher Training." Learning and Skills Development Agency. Accessed March 15, 2013. http://dera.ioe.ac.uk/10390/1/Recollected%2520in%2520tran quility.pdf

HEA (Higher Education Academy). 2011. "The UK Professional Standards Framework for Teaching and Supporting Learning in Higher Education." Accessed April 2, 2013. https://www.heacademy.ac.uk/sites/default/files/downloads/UKPSF_2011_English.pdf

Holley, D., and M. Oliver. 2010. "Student Engagement and Blended Learning: Portraits of Risk." *Computers & Education* 54 (3): 693–700.

Hramiak, A. 2010. "Online Learning Community Development with Teachers as a Means of Enhancing Initial Teacher Training." *Journal of Technology, Pedagogy and Education* 19 (1): 47–62.

Hughes, G. 2007. "Using Blended Learning to Increase Learner Support and Improve Retention." *Teaching in Higher Education* 12 (3): 349–363.

Husband, G. 2012. "Case Study: Models of Teacher Training in Further Education." Report for Edinburgh College of Further Education, Edinburgh, UK.

Independent Review Panel. 2012. "Professionalism in Further Education." Interim report for the Minister of State for Further Education, Skills and Lifelong Learning. Accessed March 10, 2013. https://www.gov.uk/government/uploads/system/uploads/attachment_data/file/422229/bis-12-670-professionalism-in-further-education-review-interim-report.pdf

Ingleby, E. 2011. "Asclepius or Hippocrates? Differing Interpretations of Post-compulsory Initial Teacher Training Mentoring." *Journal of Vocational Education & Training* 63 (1): 15–25.

Khoo, E., M. Forret, and B. Cowie, eds. 2009. "Developing an Online Learning Community: A Model for Enhancing Lecturer and Student Learning Experiences." In *Same Places, Different Spaces*. Proceedings of Ascilite Auckland, 2009. Accessed April 4, 2013. http://www.ascilite.org.au/conferences/auckland09/procs/khoo.pdf

Laurillard, D. 2008. "Digital Technologies and Their Role in Achieving Our Ambitions for Education." Inaugural lecture to Institute of Education, University of London. Accessed March 15, 2013. http://eprints.ioe.ac.uk/628/1/Laurillard2008Digital_technologies.pdf

Lave, J., and E. Wenger. 2002. "Legitimate Peripheral Participation in Communities of Practice." In *Supporting Lifelong Learning, Volume 1, Perspectives on Learning*, edited by J. C. R. Harrison, F. Reeve, and A. Hanson, 111–126. London: Routledge.

Lea, S., and L. Callaghan. 2006. "Lecturers on Teaching in the 'Supercomplexity' of Higher Education." *Higher Education* 55 (2): 171–187.

Lucas, N., and L. Unwin. 2009. "Developing Teacher Expertise at Work: Inservice Trainee Teachers in Colleges of Further Education in England." *Journal of Further and Higher Education* 33 (4): 423–433.

Lueger, M., and O. Vettori. 2008. "'Flexibilising' Standards? The Role of Quality Standards within a Participative Quality Culture." In *Implementing and Using Quality Assurance: Strategy and Practice*, 11–17. Proceedings of 2nd European Quality Assurance Forum. Brussels, Belgium: European University Association.

Mason, J. 2002. *Qualitative Researching*. 2nd ed. London: Sage.

Mathews, D. 2013. "Degrees of Comparability." *Times Higher Education*. Accessed March 28, 2013. www.timeshighereducation.co.uk

Mutton, T., G. Mills, and J. McNicholl. 2006. "Mentor Skills in a New Context: Working with Trainee Teachers to Develop the Use of Information and Communications Technology in Their Subject Teaching." *Journal of Technology, Pedagogy and Education* 15 (3): 337–352.

Nwabude, A., and G. Ade-Ojo. 2008. "Changing Times, Changing Roles: FE Colleges' Perceptions of Their Changing Leadership Role in Contemporary UK Politico-Economic Climate." In *X BCES Conference International Perspectives on Education*, 199–205. Sofia, Bulgaria: Bulgarian Comparative Education Society.

O'Leary, M. 2013. "Expansive and Restrictive Approaches to Professionalism in FE Colleges: The Observation of Teaching and Learning as a Case in Point." *Research in Post-Compulsory Education* 18 (4): 348–364.

Orr, K. 2010. "The Entry of 14–16 Year Old Students into Colleges: Implications for Further Education Initial Teacher Training in England." *Journal of Further and Higher Education* 34 (1): 47–57.

Orvis, K., R. Brusso, M. Wasserman, and S. Fisher. 2010. "E-Nabled for E-Learning? The Moderating Role of Personality in Determining the Optimal Degree of Learner Control in an E-Learning Environment." *Journal of Human Performance* 24 (1): 60–78.

Parsons, D., I. Hill, J. Holland, and D. Willis. 2012. *Impact of Teaching Development Programmes in Higher Education*. York, UK: The Higher Education Academy.

Saldana, J. 2011. *Fundamentals of Qualitative Research*. Oxford: Oxford University Press.

Scandura, T., M. Tejeda, W. Werther, M. Lankau, and C. Gables. 1996. "Perspectives on Mentoring." *Leadership and Organization Development Journal* 17 (3): 50–56.

Simmons, R. 2008. "Golden Years? Further Education Colleges under Local Authority Control." *Journal of Further and Higher Education* 32 (4): 359–371.

Skills Commission. 2010. *Teacher Training in Vocational Education*. London: Skills Commission.

Spenceley, L. 2012. "'The Odd Couple': An FE Educator's Perspective of the Management of Behaviour of 'Special Needs' Learners in the Lifelong Learning Sector." *Research in Post-Compulsory Education* 17 (3): 311–320.

Svensson, G., and G. Wood. 2007. "Are University Students Really Customers? When Illusion May Lead to Delusion for All!" *International Journal of Educational Management* 21 (1): 17–28.

Thody, A. 2006. *Writing and Presenting Research*. London: Sage.

Valenčič, M., and J. Vogrinc. 2007. "A Mentor's Aid in Developing the Competences of Teacher Trainees." *Journal of Educational Studies* 33 (4): 373–384.

Wend, P. 2013. "What Are Universities for?" In *Proceedings of The International Partners' Conference 2013*, 30–43. Accessed April 5, 2013. http://www.regents.ac.uk/media/53027/draft2_ipo_proceedings_-_final.pdf

Wenger, E. 1998. "Communities of Practice and Social Learning Systems: The Career of a Concept." *A Social Systems View on Learning: Communities of Practice as Social Learning Systems*. Accessed April 15, 2013. http://wenger-trayner.com/wp-content/uploads/2012/01/09-10-27-CoPs-and-systems-v2.01.pdf

Wertz, F., and K. Charmaz. 2011. *Five Ways of Doing Qualitiative Analysis: Phenomenological Psychology, Grounded Theory, Discourse Analysis, Narrative Research and Intuitive Inquiry*. London: Guildford Press.

Whitchurch, C. 2008. "Shifting Identities, Blurring Boundaries: The Changing Roles of Professional Managers in Higher Education." *Centre for Studies in Higher Education* 62: 1–9.

Woodd, M. 1997. "Mentoring in Further and Higher Education: Learning from the Literature." *Journal for Education and Training* 39 (9): 333–343.

Yin, R. 2011. *Qualitative Research from Start to Finish*. Oxford: Guildford Publications.

Legislation

Further and Higher Education Act. 1992. UK Government.

Data Protection Act. 1998. UK Government.

Professional Standards for Lecturers in Scotland's Colleges. 2012. Scottish Government.

'Nothing will prevent me from doing a good job'. The professionalisation of part-time teaching staff in further and adult education

Jill Jameson and Yvonne Hillier

Approximately 85,000 part-time teaching staff working in further education (FE) and adult and community learning (ACL) are often seen as 'a problem'. The intrinsic 'part-timeness' of these staff tends to marginalise them: they remain under-recognised and largely unsupported. Yet this picture is over-simplified. This article examines how part-time staff make creative use of professional autonomy and agency to mitigate problematic 'casual employment' conditions, reporting on results from Learning and Skills Development Agency-sponsored research (2002–2006) with 700 part-time staff in the learning and skills sector. The question of agency was reported as a key factor in part-time employment. Change is necessary for the professional agency of part-timers to be harnessed as the sector responds to ambitious sectoral 'improvement' agendas following the Foster Report and FE White Paper. Enhanced professionalisation for part-time staff needs greater recognition and inclusion in change agendas.

Introduction

Approximately 85,000 part-time teaching staff who work in further education (FE) and adult and community learning (ACL) are often seen as 'a problem'. By the very nature of their part-timeness, they are not able to participate in team meetings, staff development, or to be on hand to discuss issues in the professional practice of teaching and learning with full-time colleagues. In order to carry out their valuable, demanding part-time work on the various slippery 'edges' of institutions funded by the Learning and Skills Council (LSC), part-time staff overcome problems in many ways, often juggling and managing their roles with highly developed levels of professional expertise. They remain under-recognised and largely unsupported by institutions. They almost invariably have significantly less access than full-time staff to professional recognition, management support, teaching and learning resources, staff development, communication and even basic classroom and canteen facilities. They tend to lack appropriate pay, quality support and curriculum training (NATFHE 2001, 2005). They are usually relegated to subordinate, marginalised positions in the hierarchies of institutions, while simultaneously being overloaded with inappropriately burdensome administrative demands. They are even sometimes scapegoated as 'the reason' why some institutions provide less than satisfactory learning opportunities. Yet this picture is over simplified and inaccurate (Hillier and Jameson 2004, 2006).

Change is necessary if part-timers are to contribute to the ambitious agenda for change and quality improvement now on the horizon of implementation during 2006–2010 following the Foster Report (DfES/LSC 2005), Leitch Review of Skills (HM Treasury 2006) and the government Reform White Paper on FE (2006). This article examines how part-time staff currently make unexpectedly *eudaemonic* (i.e. joyful) use of their professional autonomy and agency to mitigate the problems of being in casual employment, reporting on the results of Learning and Skills Development Agency (LSDA)-sponsored research carried out with part-time staff in the learning and skills sector (LSS), in which the question of agency was reported as a key factor in the employment of part-time staff. The paper asks how such agency can be harnessed, particularly as the sector responds to the proposals of the Foster Report (DfES/LSC 2005) and the FE White Paper (2006). It argues that the Institute for Learning (IfL) can play a key role in ensuring that this dedicated group of staff in further and adult education is not only included in the demanding and ambitious agenda for change in the sector but is regarded as central to it.

This article makes recommendations on the way in which experiences of part-time staff need to be understood by leaders and managers in FE at a time when a spate of new policies concerning workforce development, to meet both institutional targets and the aspirations of learners, will come into force following the FE White Paper. We describe how we undertook an examination of part-time staff in FE and ACL in 2002–2006 using a model of practitioner research developed by the Learning and Skills Research Network London and South East (LSRN LSE), funded by the then LSDA.

An overwhelmed sector

In 2003, the authors argued that it had been 'raining policy' in FE for many years (Hillier and Jameson 2003), recommending ways in which those faced with continuous top-down change could respond effectively and proactively while retaining their autonomy (Jameson and Hillier 2003). Insistent rain has subsequently turned into a torrent of apparently unending top-down educational policy changes and developments. Although FE and ACL provision is high on the governmental menu of educational priorities in relation to skills and economic agendas, this brings considerably increased pressures as well. The increasing emphasis on 'skills' in government policy, combined with budgetary cuts to adult education, has also created great uncertainty regarding continuity of funding for non-vocational FE and adult education: nationally, the numbers of adult education students have in consequence been rapidly declining. All of these issues impact on part-time staff in FE and adult education institutions. The torrent of policy initiatives and the outfall resulting from them means that part-time staff working in large numbers at these slippery, vulnerable edges of the LSS are increasingly at risk of falling off altogether.

The national significance of the issues involved

Further and adult education form a substantial part of the UK national LSS, which, overall, is huge. The national budget for the LSC in 2004/05 was £9.2 billion, of which £5.1 billion (54.9%) was spent on young people and £2.9 billion (32.5%) on adults. FE institutions received a budget nationally of £4.4933 billion (48.6%). In the same period, around six million people participated in LSC-funded education and training (LSC 2005b, 2–3). The LSC (LSC 2005b, 22–23) reported that in the two years to 2003/04, success rates in FE colleges rose from 65% to 72%, with learners achieving 350,000 additional qualifications (LSC 2005b, 22–23). These achievements indicate that institutions and individuals throughout the LSS sector worked ever harder to enable learners to achieve their goals. Although the number of FE colleges in 2005 declined from 435 to 382 nationally as result of mergers and closures (LSC 2005a), the FE/ACL sub-sector is now relatively healthy financially and there is a continuing imperative for it to 'deliver' on skills, learning achievements, quality improvement and social inclusion. The sector has, in short, a critically important national UK-wide role to play.

Since 2002, multiple simultaneous 14–19 and adult policy developments have been launched, including curriculum, leadership and management initiatives, quality improvements, social inclusion agendas, skills and employment initiatives, children's services multi-agency developments, adult basic skills agendas, beacon institution awards, schools' trust, city academy initiatives, changes to the structure of 14–19 and adult qualifications, new partnerships, e-learning developments and major reforms of educational provision. In short, there has been an unstoppable deluge of reforming agendas from 2002 within which everyone, employed either part-time or full-time in the learning and skills system, has been caught up (Hillier 2006; Jameson and McNay 2007). Some of the main policy initiatives are outlined briefly below and then discussed in relation to the ways in which these affect part-time staff.

Policy developments affecting part-time staff

Following the publication of *Success for All* (DfES 2002), an unprecedented period of policy changes and developments occurred in learning and skills, focusing on skills and qualifications. The original skills strategy White Paper, *21st Century Skills: Realising our Potential* (DfES 2003a), was updated in March 2005 as a new Skills White Paper, *Skills: Getting on in Business, Getting on at Work* (DfES 2005b). Simultaneously, widespread increased investments in FE were aimed at additional programmes to meet the needs of adults without basic skills in a Level 2 entitlement, to be implemented from 2006/07. The updated Skills for Life Strategy was produced in 2003 (DfES 2003b), outlining a new strategy for basic skills development. These areas have traditionally been taught primarily by part-time staff, who have been faced with the necessity of responding very quickly and very often to wide scale qualifications, curriculum and other government-imposed changes.

In February 2005, the government published the 14–19 White Paper (DfES 2005a), confirming the LSC's central role in providing education and skills for young people. In the same year, the highest ever number of young people in education and training was recorded in England. In March 2005 the Chancellor pledged an extra £350 million for investment in FE buildings for 2008–2010 and the Skills White Paper (DfES 2005b), outlined anticipated skill needs for businesses and adults. A major DfES/LSC-commissioned review of the future role of FE, the Foster Review (DfES/LSC 2005), was finalised during 2005, with its results reported and follow-up work already under way. A Treasury-sponsored report from the Review of Skills project team led by Lord Leitch on skills needs and identifiable gaps for the next 15 years until 2020 was commissioned (HM Treasury 2005, 2006). During this period, also, the NIACE report *Eight in Ten* (NIACE 2005), on the state of adult learning in FE, was produced, and *Train to Gain*, the national roll-out of the employer training pilots, was implemented: all areas in which staffing by part-timers is a noticeable feature.

The Foster Review stressed the importance of FE, noting that its potential is as yet insufficiently recognised. It recommended that the future focus of FE should be on skills, with 'values of greater clarity, improved leadership, organisation and management and a relentless focus on the needs of learners and business as the criteria for progress' (DfES/LSC 2005). The report observed that FE colleges had achieved many things effectively, but also noted that 'there are many symptoms indicating all is not well'.

Selected key recommendations from the review included the proposals that FE colleges needed clearer purposes, notably the three main functions of: building vocational skills, promoting social inclusion and achieving academic progress. The Foster Review Team recommended that FE should concentrate mainly on supplying skills, vocational learning and employability for learners in ways useful for the UK economy, and that the FE system's role in promoting social inclusion was also important and should be retained. In addition, the team reported that the drive to improve quality must continue and is vital to achieve the core purposes of FE (DfES/LSC 2005).

Of immediate direct relevance to part-time staff is the Foster Review's recognition that the 'increasingly "casualised" and ageing nature of the workforce' in FE needs to be tackled, and that 'pedagogic and vocational skills need to improve through comprehensive workforce planning and development'. Furthermore, Foster recognised that, 'Morale is low at present and there are staff retention problems' in FE (DfES/LSC 2005). The sense of low morale and feelings of relative powerlessness on the part of the workforce to change conditions in the sector were also reported by the Economic and Social Research Council's (ESRC's) large-scale research project – the Transforming Learning Cultures project, in which it was discovered that tutors were spending their time protecting the existing learning culture from 'external damage' and that 'amounts of "underground" working' occurred whereby tutors routinely engaged in working well beyond their job descriptions. The report argued that tutors were 'running out of the energy and morale' needed to mediate national managerialist approaches (TLRP 2005).

In this climate, the government Reform White Paper *Further Education, Raising Skills, Improving Life Chances* (2006) put in place the requirement that all new staff in FE must gain a new teaching qualification from 2007. This new qualification will provide qualified tutor, learning and skills status, a licence to practice based upon new professional standards to be created by Lifelong Learning UK (LLUK), the Sector Skills Council for learning in FE, ACL and work-based learning. In addition, staff will be required to undertake continuing professional development (CPD) to maintain their licence to practice.

Impact of policy on part-time staff and legislation

The impact of the above policies on part-time staff is affected by another important piece of legislation. The LSS must implement the Part-time Workers (Prevention of Less Favourable Treatment) Regulations 2000 which came into force on 1 July, 2000. These regulations implemented the European Directive on the Framework Agreement on Part-time Work (97/81/EC, amended by Directive 98/23/EC). The 2000 regulations on part-time workers aim to eliminate discrimination against part-timers and to improve the quality of their work. Since 2000, part-time staff should not have been treated in a less favourable way solely because they work part-time unless there was an objective justification for differential treatment. This key legislation underpins the argument for parity with full-time staff. It is increasingly important for employers at all levels to abide by the terms of the legislation. In the longer-term, part-timers will benefit from changing conditions following the implementation of these regulations more effectively in future years across the LSS. In the short-term, however, colleges reeling from the above glut of policy changes and the reduction of funding for non-vocational education may be tempted to cut costs by overloading and neglecting existing part-timers, saving staffing funds by cutting courses and generally continuing to marginalise part-time staff in terms of parity with full-timers for curriculum support, funding, learning resources and management time.

The policy context in which people must work in FE is incomplete without addressing the action undertaken by the part-time staff themselves, however. Notions of professionalism and the ways in which these affect the responses by staff to policy initiatives provide an important interplay of forces. The cultural and professional environment affecting those who work in FE needs further examination.

Managerialism and the 'audit culture' in the LSS

Many post-compulsory education institutions appear to foster, deliberately or not, a performative task-focused environment in which relatively more or less coercive managerial behaviour is the norm to enforce target-setting and compliance among staff in meeting those targets. A recent on-line survey of leadership in the LSS carried out in 2006–2007 (Jameson and McNay 2007) collected 191 responses overall, from which 85 respondents from FE, adult education and other LSC-funded post-16 institutions described the organisation they worked for according to Blake and Mouton's (1978) four profiles for management (in which management are described as having concerns [or not] for people, tasks and/or teams). The largest percentage of respondents to this question (36%, 31 respondents) in mixed survey LSS results including both managers and academic staff selected the description 'authority-compliance management – high concern for task, but low concern for people' for their LSS institutions. There were, overall, 35 people in FE and adult education who replied that their institutions were either managed through 'authority-compliance' or could be characterised by the description, 'impoverished management – low concern for both tasks and people' (four respondents). Responses from full-time (n=15) and part-time (n=3) lecturing staff in LSS institutions (n=18) indicated that 61% (11 respondents) felt that the culture in their institutions was either one of 'authority compliance' management (nine respondents) or 'impoverished management' (two respondents) with one part-time FE college staff member expressing serious concerns about the degree of 'bullying and dictatorial' management. Another part-time staff respondent from an FE college wrote, in 2007, that management in the college:

> ...are only interested in the financial well being of the college and of achieving good Ofsted results. They do not take the time to see what is going on at the chalk face and only pay lip service at informing teachers and middle management of decisions taken... They do not consult on matters that affect staff or students and do not demonstrate an understanding of issues which affect staff... colleagues were upset that the SMT member didn't even know how many classes are held on our site and suggestions for improvement showed no understanding of the issues involved.

> (see also Jameson and McNay 2007)

Market-led funding principles under the former Further Education Funding Council helped to create an increasingly business-focused climate following the incorporation of colleges in 1992/93 (Ainley and Bailey 1997; Elliott 1996; Goddard-Patel and Whitehead 2000). In 2002, Avis noted that FE was marked by the:

> ...growth of managerialism following incorporation... funding was prioritised. The need to operate institutions with a declining level of resource led to the pursuit of efficiency gains which in turn encouraged the development of an abrasive managerial culture concerned with increasing the effectiveness of the labour power at its disposal.

> (Avis 2002, 344)

A relatively strict differentiation between 'senior management', 'middle management' and 'staff' consequently developed in many post-compulsory institutions, in which an allegedly powerful masculinist culture (Kerfoot and Whitehead 1998; Shain 1999, 2000) thrived, to the detriment of staff committed to collegiate professionalism and equity. This 'managerialist' culture (Randle and Brady 1997) regards lecturers not so much as equals but as subordinates occupying 'follower' positions. The tendency for managers involved in corporate compliance to try to control their staff does not sit well with practitioner staff in FE, who in many cases regard themselves as hard-working 'professionals' and do not take kindly to over-zealous control by managers.

Part-time staff who work in this environment are deeply affected by policy at every level, whether directly or indirectly. Such staff are, however, situated on the 'outer edges' of LSC-funded institutions and therefore not as bound in by the relentless targets of the prevailing 'audit culture' in which both part-time and full-time staff are working in an environment increasingly scrutinised by a range of agencies. The fact that part-time staff are more or less at the margins of this culture simultaneously endows them with desirable freedoms and regrettable insecurities, as well as problems with implementing successful learning and teaching.

Professionalism of FE staff

In the context of the wider literature on professionalism (Downie 1990; Frowe 2005), a growing literature debating the concept of professionalism in post-compulsory education (Randle and Brady 1997; Avis 2002; Hyland and Merrill 2003; Avis and Bathmaker 2004; Spenceley 2006) has recorded many concerns about the relative lack of status of teaching staff as professionals. The problematic status of 'professionalism' within the LSS teaching workforce, both academic and vocational, in particular in FE, is well recognised. Clow (2001) analysed a number of different strands of 'professionalism' identifiable and potentially applicable to FE teachers, in terms of the history of 'professionalism' and the hallmarks of what constitutes a 'profession', concluding that:

> It is no great surprise that the diversity of FE produces a diversity of constructions of professionalism… It is argued that a cohesive view of professionalism could create a less exploited workforce and lead to an improved quality of teaching in FE.

> (Clow 2001, 407)

Clow (2001) builds on an earlier study on FE by Robson (1998), who had drawn attention to the difficulties of conceptualising 'professionalism' effectively within FE. Robson observed that although the identity of the FE sector as a whole had been advanced by the implementation of the Further and Higher Education Act 1992, FE teachers had not enjoyed concomitant benefits regarding enhanced recognition of professional status. In fact, Robson noted that:

> The current crisis in the further education sector has highlighted that professional group's marginality and low status… The FE teaching profession… lacks closure and is not clearly demarcated… Though some possibilities may exist within certain 'managerialist' initiatives, real change will require major legislative and policy shifts, as well as a full reappraisal of the sector's funding.

> (Robson 1998, 585)

Spenceley (2006) updates this debate and takes it into new directions to examine the 'smoke and mirrors' of a looking glass world which reflects the rhetoric of FE professionalism. Spenceley reinforces the concept that FE lecturing staff as a whole are relatively 'vulnerable' in terms of professionalism (Spenceley 2006). The 'lack of closure' and 'demarcation' of FE teaching as a profession is arguably felt by most teaching staff. This situation is, however, particularly acute in the case of part-time lecturers, in view of their institutional vulnerability and marginalisation. Earlier work by Randle and Brady (1997) outlines a basic tension between 'managerialism' on the one hand, and 'professionalism' on the other. This tension is notably likely to be more strained when professional staff are part-time and therefore more distant from structural institutional hierarchies.

Having discussed the general problems of defining 'professionalism', Downie (1990) proposed that professionals could be characterised by the possession of expertise within a broad knowledge base, by relationships of integrity and service to clients authorised by a professional body, by the social function of speaking out on behalf of a profession, by independence from state or commercial interests and by the fact that they are 'educated' in a broad sense, rather than merely 'trained'. These professional characteristics, as applied to FE, are encapsulated by Robson (2006) into three basic constituents of professionalism: autonomy, professional knowledge and responsibility. She argues that the notion of any occupation holding fixed, unchangeable defining characteristics is both unhelpful and lacks credibility. Her discussion of autonomy acknowledges that it is the reduction of teacher autonomy in recent years that has 'stirred feelings like no other' (Robson 2006, 11). Ollin also notes the resulting 'culture of victimhood' so often expressed by teachers who feel increasingly powerless against the progressively more centralised control of their work (Ollin 2005, 151). She draws upon previous work (Avis 1999) which identifies that teachers can be represented as being 'powerless victims of forces beyond their control' (Ollin 2005, 152). Ollin's conceptualisation of professionalism includes action by individuals to protect professional standards, such as resistance to practical changes affecting work practices, resisting change implementation and a more overall ideological resistance. She argues that, for each of these, action should be taken at micro and macro levels and that action at the micro-level is particularly significant in subverting or undermining large-scale structures. This notion of individual action, even at micro-level, is interesting when examined in the context of casual staff, as explored later in this article.

Activity systems

One way to examine the different perspectives arising from the tension between 'managerialism' and 'professionalism' is to apply activity theory to this complex area of practice. As Avis (2002) note, FE teachers should be conceptualised within the context of activity theory in which they are part of a set of relationships or activity systems (see Engestrom 1987, 2001). Interactive systems theories take account of the history and biography of individuals in systems and examine these to help explain the meaning of their actions. For example, in FE and ACL there are *trajectories* of the institution (the paths followed by the institution), as well as trajectories followed by the department, by course teams, and also individual trajectories of part-time staff who are teaching on courses. These are loosely linked, but they do not necessarily follow the same trajectory. Contradictions and tensions within the activity system are acknowledged in interactive systems analysis. Casual staff, for example, experience tensions in the same way as their full-time colleagues but, in addition, they are affected by other tensions that need to be managed, particularly if such staff work in isolation from their full time peers, perhaps off site or outside day-time provision.

Professionals can be at loggerheads with attempts by managers within institutions to control them, as the very definition of 'professional' implies a degree of self-controlled autonomy within a community of practice which is wider than any one institution. Lave and Wenger (1991) define such a community as:

> A set of relations among persons, activity and world, over time and in relation with other tangential and overlapping communities of practice
>
> (Lave and Wenger 1991, 98)

Such relations typically require high levels of trust, and sustained evolutionary development within the work-related and social interactions of a group of professionals who meet together face-to-face and also correspond through online and telephone communications. In their research into the experiences of new entrants to FE, Bathmaker and Avis (2005) identified that marginalisation can be related to the impact of current changes in FE, notably, 'poor workplace conditions, lack of resources, perceived lack of management support' which affects communities of practice and therefore leads to 'low morale, being burnt out and having lost commitment to students' (61). They found that new trainees in FE can be marginalised from the *legitimate* peripheral participation that Lave and Wenger (2002) describe, whereby it is expected that new entrants to FE teaching would have fewer demands placed on them than their full-time counterparts. Yet access to the community of practice is vital if newcomers are to learn from each other. This paper argues that part-timers also experience marginalisation from what may be seen as an acceptable level of legitimate peripheral participation. Nevertheless, interestingly, part-time staff who are part of communities of practice as autonomous professionals also seem, ironically. to be somewhat liberated by their very *part-timeness* from being locked into patterns of control and de-professionalisation by management in institutions. They have, in other words, some desirable freedoms.

Given the tensions outlined above for anyone working in FE in the present climate, this paper examines evidence regarding the experiences of those who are hourly paid or fractional.

Method

Examining the deployment of part-time staff in FE

The 2002/03 LSDA-funded research project investigated part-time staff deployment and development in the LSS. Statistical analysis of 700 questionnaires and follow-up interviews was undertaken by college researchers working in four FE colleges and one adult education service in London and the South East (Hillier and Jameson 2004). The analysis highlighted the enthusiasm, professionalism and commitment of part-time staff but also their frustration, lack of support and status at work when compared with full-time colleagues. We argued that part-time staff were insecurely situated at the margins of institutions, despite the important contributions they made to the sector as a result of their work on the curriculum and the overall quality of their work. This led us to apply the term 'ragged trousered philanthropy', building on Tressell's original conception (Tressell 1993[1914]) to capture the way in which part-time staff undertook 'good works' for relatively low wages and poor conditions. We argued then that institutions could not and should not over-rely on the good will of part-time staff to sustain working situations in which institutional employment conditions for part-timers were relatively poor.

Funding was obtained by LSDA in 2005/06 to carry out a further analysis of the unexpectedly rich qualitative data that had emerged from the questionnaires and interviews. Coding of the original 700 questionnaires was carried out using Atlas-Ti software for qualitative analysis. Using a grounded theory approach, the team created a series of codes from the original data, applying an extended analysis to test the findings of the 2004 report.

Qualitative data analysis of questionnaires

The open-ended questionnaire items listed below (see Table 1) yielded the qualitative data analysed in the 2002–2004 and 2005–2006 projects:

Table 1.   Selected questions from LSDA-funded LSRN LSE part-time staff research, 2002–2006.

Questions in the Part-time Staff Survey

Q3c: *Are there any comments that you would like to make concerning what your pay covers? What staff development opportunities or changes in staff development organisation would help you in your role?*

Q8: *In this institution, do you have the following kinds of support from these staff (your line manager, part-time colleagues, full-time colleagues: e.g. induction, information/materials, observation and feedback on teaching, mentoring, staff development, opportunities to share problems with others, attend social events, access to support from trade union, staff association)?*

Q9: *What resources that you don't have would help to improve your teaching? Are these available to full-time colleagues?*

Q11a and b: *Have you discussed your resources needs with anyone at your institution? If 'Yes', with whom?*

Q13: *What levels of support do you get from your line manager and colleagues?*

Q14: *Please list the features of your employment that enable you to do a good job.*

Q15: *Please list the features of your employment that prevent you doing a good job*

Table 2.   Codes emerging from qualitative data: LSDA-funded LSRN part-time staff Research 2005–2006.

• accommodation	• level of connection
• administration	• line manager support
• autonomy	• management
• communication	• positive view
• comparison with full-time staff	• views of teaching
• curriculum manager	• quotable
• discontent	• teaching equipment
• enthusiasm	• teaching resources and curriculum guidance
• ethos	• team meetings and liaison
• experience	• using own resources
• individual agency	• valued
• insecurity	• view of rate of pay

Approximately 300 codes were derived from an extensive analysis of questionnaire data from part-time staff respondents using Atlas-Ti. Some codes related to case study sites contributing location-specific information to overall conceptual analysis. Following the initial analysis, all codes were subsequently regrouped into more extensive codes. These were analysed in the context of part-timers' work in lifelong learning institutions until a saturation point was reached and all codes seemed to have been exhaustively teased out. Of these, 24 codes were identified as being important, as they were particularly frequently applied to the data, or because they represented strongly polarised views and were worth exploring in more detail. These codes are illustrated in Table 2.

An invited expert seminar group was asked to discuss and ratify the primary codes and themes in 2005–2006. The seminar group involved participants from the LSC sector, the National Institute of Adult Continuing Education (NIACE), LLUK, the National Association of Teachers in Further and Higher Education (NATFHE) and the LSDA. The expert group included a number of key individuals with extensive experience of issues relating to part-time staff in the LSS. This team discussed the issues involved in, and the impact of, the first research report on part-time staff. They made a number of recommendations. A follow-up online survey to the expert team using a questionnaire on the website www.surveymonkey.com consolidated the results of the expert team discussions, supplementing observers' notes with individual written commentary (Hillier and Jameson 2004).

The secondary analysis emerging from the data comprised the following themes:

- management
- resources including pay
- professionalism
- agency
- staff development and support
- ethos

Two of these themes, *professionalism* and *agency*, emerged as particularly pertinent to the way in which part-time staff were then, and still, are managing their working lives in the complex interactions that activity theory outlines.

Discussion

Professionalism

Evidence from the questionnaire responses can be aligned to two of the three constitutive ideas of Robson's model of professionalism: autonomy and responsibility. As noted above, tensions exist between the interactions of personal understandings and actions within the complex system of FE.

Autonomy

The following quotes demonstrate a view that, in addition to the considerable difficulties experienced by part-time staff working in the sector, there is, despite this, evidence that part-time staff experience professional benefits which relate to trust, freedom and independence. These are powerful values which Robson also identified as central to notions of what professionalism means for staff in FE. Selected respondents from the research project on part-time staff said:

- I am given scope for development and initiative. I am trusted to be professional/good

- Freedom to teach in own way

- Allowed to teach without being told what I should do – trusting atmosphere

- Being left alone to get on with it!

- Every one is concerned for and helpful to my students. THEY LET ME GET ON WITH THE JOB!!!

- My courses are flexible with plenty of scope to tailor syllabuses to individual learners needs. I am given freedom to do this.

The relationship part-time staff reported that their experience with management is interesting in relation to autonomy. The next quote from a part-time lecturer shows the way in which management is not necessarily viewed as being important or helpful:

Generally good atmosphere to work in. Mostly lack of interference from line manager (left to be autonomous)

Autonomy was also linked to notions of being student-centred and also of providing good quality teaching and learning:

- Having taught the subjects for as long as I have, the fact that I am left to plan the areas in which I teach enables me to carry out first class teaching.

- Being allowed to construct and teach my yoga course in the way I choose and judge to be appropriate for the students

- I teach out. I am professionally qualified, my courses are generally over-subscribed and I have an excellent rapport with my students. I seldom need help and like to think that I have good admin back-up but 'at a distance'! i.e. photocopying and the occasional VDU is all I require!

Professional knowledge, too, is contained within the notion of autonomy. This quote also shows the advantages of being part-time compared with full-time colleagues:

…freedom to teach aspects of the subject that I know about from the industry, that full time teachers may not cover.

Responsibility

Robson (2006, 20) had argued that it is not surprising to find that teachers in FE feel most responsible, in the first instance, to their learners (Shain and Gleeson 1999; Clow 2001). This sense of responsibility, coupled with the deep adherence to desire for autonomy, can be seen emerging from the data collected. It provides important evidence that part-time staff are both grappling with and manifesting the tensions that are bound to arise from trying to enact a professional stance to practice in the context of constraint and compliance. It is the day-to-day management of these tensions that can be seen through the notion of individual agency. In some of the positive situations reported, practitioners not only felt responsible for their learners but also took 'self-governing' action with learners at the forefront of professional practice. This sense of autonomous accountability and responsibility for the course and their learners meant part-timers shouldered burdens in the same way as if they worked independently from any institution:

- Relatively independent and self governing. Allowed to get on with it. Colleagues and managers willing to listen to my ideas. Good working atmosphere.

- If I take personal responsibility for my work and actions there are no major hindrances

- I do a good job, because I feel that I am responsible for the course, not other people

Agency

Agency relates to people's action in the world but cannot be divorced from structure, or the environment within which people live. Part-time staff are near the bottom of the hierarchical staffing structure in further and adult education. However, they may bring with them social capital from their positions in society which may help explain why some of the respondents were very active in obtaining the necessary resources, human and physical, to ensure that their learners had good quality experiences. There is a complex interaction between individual agency and management particularly discernible in this data regarding relationships with line managers, who were often but not exclusively the first 'official' institutional port of call for part-time staff. In most cases, there were good, positive responses in response to the question regarding relationship with line managers. However, as the following section shows, this is tempered with the 'busy-ness' of all staff working in the institution, and the need for individuals to take action themselves to deal with this situation:

- Contact with my line manager with time to discuss any issues or problems which also includes guidance and support and how to approach certain situations concerning students. This is mainly instigated by myself.

- I always feel they will help me if I ask. However, all the staff are usually flat out, so sometimes it is a case of help yourself!

- I do everything myself. They leave me to get on with it. But I fear they're too busy

- Probably best to say where I work is a well-meaning but pretty ineffective shambles. Accept this and everything seems okay. You're on your own. Don't expect praise. Be the best teacher you can.

- Any support I need, I have to ask for

Not all respondents demonstrated satisfaction with the degree of autonomy they experienced, and an ability to handle this in professional and proactive ways. For example, one respondent stated:

Not sure who my line manager is!!

The overall responsibilities of professionals include the requirement for staff to find out who their line manager is and to keep abreast of developments within the institution. Hence, the fact that this respondent was implicitly blaming the institution and line manager for not contacting him/her can be interpreted, to some extent, as some degree of derogation by the part-timer of her/his own professional duty. If staff are generally under-supported, there can be a risk of declining morale, feelings of resentment and rising fears of de-professionalisation which can escalate into somewhat self-destructive forms of quiet rebellion. The problem with under-resourced part-time staff situations can be that, if both line managers and part-timers are too busy or overloaded with other work to make contact with each other, both sides can be left 'blaming' the other for neglect, while the students and often the part-time staff themselves are the ones who suffer in the long run from these gaps in communication.

Despite the challenges of working in an environment which is 'busy' (though not necessarily uniquely so to part-time staff) the following quote suggests that there is a deep seated tendency within the profession to 'put learners first'. A genuine over-riding concern to do a 'good job' for learners can overcome many of the difficulties that part-time staff experience in other ways, including a lack of resources, cooperation and support:

> Total lack of co-operation from full-time teachers. Necessary equipment always difficult to use as either hidden beneath piles of cardboard, and/or usually messy and dirty after day classes. However, I always manage to do a 'good job' for my students regardless.

Perhaps the last word should rest with one part-time respondent who argued the following:

> Nothing will prevent me from doing a good job.

There is, within this self-defined declaration of adherence to professional standards, a sense of eudaemonic well-being fostered within the part-time margins of further and adult education institutions. This is relentlessly maintained in spite of the considerable difficulties and problems of experiencing the state of part-timeness within the sector. In this, part-time staff members protect and celebrate unexpected freedoms to determine autonomously their own professional high standards of good quality in teaching and learning. Institutions and sectoral agencies can learn much from the resolute adherence of such staff to high professional standards in despite of every obstacle.

Harnessing the professional agency and autonomy of part-timers for good

There is an important challenge facing all who work within or relating to the FE sector. An overwhelmingly casualised workforce is still marginalised by government policy: the requirement for staff to hold teaching qualifications and to undertake CPD from September 2007 has yet to specify how part-time staff can be supported by their institutions. There are implications for the management and leadership of part-time staff: the role of the Centre for Excellence in Leadership and the IfL will be crucial to help foster appropriate ways in which to support part-time staff.

The IfL: opportunities and challenges

The IfL response to the White Paper *Further Education, Raising Skills, Improving Life Chances* (IfL 2006) specifically addressed the way in which teachers in FE can continually improve their practice through CPD. In an appendix to this response, IfL outlined its Code of Professional Values and Practices. Amongst the values, the following claims are made:

> Change is endemic in teaching: the role of the teacher is extremely diverse and changes over time, reflecting the developing interests of the teacher, the changing nature of learners and the influence of external policy on professional practice. Teachers highly regard the benefits of working in peer teams and in partnership with external groups such as employers, parents, community groups and related agencies. Collegiality and collaboration ensures the relevance and responsiveness of learning programmes and facilitates the sharing of best practice.

(IfL 2006, 15)

The marginalisation of casual hourly paid as well as more permanent part-time staff constrains just how much collegiality and collaboration is possible for part-timers, especially those over-burdened by pressures on time from split-site work/travel to fulfil several different part-time jobs. It is, however, unhelpful to ignore the institutional working contexts of hourly-paid staff. A network such as the IfL affords the potential for part-timers to participate in an on-going community of professional practice if they are unable to attend routine programme meetings or professional development activities. To offer opportunities to update professional knowledge about new initiatives and to share experiences online using asynchronous virtual access is a key strand of IfL's planned activities and is to be welcomed. However, institutions do also need to provide necessary support for and the inclusion of casual and part-time staff in events, meetings and other forums, including online communications, newsletter and staff development activities, if part-time staff are to be enabled to feel included as part of the community of practice of teachers in FE.

Conclusion

The data and analysis reported from this two-phase LSDA-funded research project on part-time staff (2002–2006) indicate that there is enormous potential and energy which can be harnessed by institutions if they are to recognise the autonomy, responsibility and personal agency which reside in their part-time staff. Hourly-paid and fractional staff in FE and ACL make enormous efforts to protect their learners from poor quality provision and, freed from the managerialist traps into which many full-time staff are locked, make unexpectedly *eudaemonic* use of their freedoms to be self-defined as 'professionals'. It is the responsibility of managers and leaders in the sector to recognise the important role that is played by such staff. As James (2005) have already argued, practitioners in the sector have to manage their professionalism in a complex environment. This research suggests that there is much to be learnt from listening to the richness and complexity of the lived experiences of this vulnerable and important group of part-time staff, and supporting the further development of their professionalism.

Acknowledgements

The authors acknowledge and thank the former LSDA and LSRN LSE for funding to support this research project investigating part-time staff in further and adult education. We thank the LSRN LSE research team for their collegiate participation in the project, all the part-time staff respondents to our questionnaires and follow-up interviews and the expert seminar group participants for their help and support. In particular, we thank Mike Cooper, Trixi Blair, Graham Knight, Lindsey Baker and the project team.

References

Ainley, P., and B. Bailey. 1997. *The business of learning.* London: Cassell.
Avis, J. 1999. Shifting identity: New conditions and the transformation of practice-teaching within post-compulsory education. *Journal of Vocational Education and Training* 51: 245–264.
———. 2002. Developing staff in further education: discourse, learners and practice. *Research in Post-Compulsory Education* 7, no. 3: 339–352.
Avis, J., and A.M. Bathmaker. 2004. The politics of care: emotional labour and trainee further education lecturers. *Journal of Vocational Education and Training* 56, no. 1: 301–306.

Bathmaker, A.-M., and J. Avis. 2005. Becoming a lecturer in further education in England: The construction of professional identity and the role of communities of practice. *Journal of Education for Teaching* 31, no. 1: 47–62.

———. 1978. *The new managerial grid*. Houston, TX: Gulf Publishing.

Clow, R. 2001. Further education teachers' constructions of professionalism. *Journal of Vocational Education and Training* 53, no. 3: 407–419.

DfES. 2002. *Success for all: reforming further education and training*. Discussion document. London: Department for Education and Skills.

———. 2003a. *21st century skills: realising our potential: individuals, employers, nation*. Cm 5810. London: Department for Education and Skills.

———. 2003b. *Skills for life: the national strategy for improving adult literacy and numeracy skills: Focus on delivery to 2007*. Nottingham, UK: DfES Publications.

———. 2005a. *14–19 education and skills*. Cm 6476. London: HMSO.

———. 2005b. *Skills: getting on in business, getting on at work*. Cm 6483. London: Department for Education and Skills.

———. 2006. *Further education: raising skills, improving life chances*. Department for education and skills, Cm 6768, March. Norwich: The Stationary Office.

DfES/LSC. 2005. *Realising the potential: a review of the future role of further education colleges* (the Foster Review). London: Department for Education and Skills/Learning and Skills Council.

Downie, R.S. 1990. Professions and professionalism. *Journal of Philosophy of Education* 24, no. 2: 147–159.

Elliott, G. 1996. Educational management and the crisis of reform in further education. *Journal of Vocational Education and Training* 48, no. 1: 5–23.

Engestrom, Y. 1987. *Learning by expanding: an activity theoretical approach to development research*. Helsinki, Finland: Orienta-Konsultit Oy.

———. 2001. Expansive learning at work: toward an activity theoretical reconceptualisation. *Journal of Education and Work* 14: 133–156

Eraut, M. 1994. *Developing professional knowledge and competence*. Lewes: Falmer

Frowe, I. 2005. Professional trust. *British Journal of Educational Studies* 53, no. 1: 34–53.

Glaser, B.G., and A.L. Strauss. 1967. *The discovery of grounded theory: strategies for qualitative research*. Chicago, IL: Aldine.

Goddard-Patel, P. and S. Whitehead. 2000. Examining the crisis of further education: An analysis of 'failing colleges and failing policies'. *Policy Studies* 21, no. 3: 191–212.

Hillier, Y., and J. Jameson. 2003. *Empowering researchers in further education*. Stoke on Trent, UK: Trentham Books.

———. 2004. *A rich contract? Or, the ragged trousered philanthropy of part-time staff*. Regional research report of the LSRN LSE. London: LSDA.

——— 2006. *Leadership in post-compulsory education: inspiring leaders of the future*. London: David Fulton Publishers, Granada Media.

Hillier, Y., and A. Thompson, eds. 2004. *Readings in post-compulsory education: research in the learning and skills sector*. London: Continuum.

HM Treasury. 2005. *Skills in the UK: The long-term challenge: Leitch review of skills interim report*. London: HM Stationery Office. http://www.hm-treasury.gov.uk/independent_reviews/leitch_review/review_leitch_index.cfm.

———. 2006. *Prosperity for all in the global economy – world class skills. Final Report December 2006*. London: HM Stationery Office

Hyland, T., and B. Merrill. 2003. *The changing face of further education: lifelong learning, inclusion and community values in further education*. London: Taylor & Francis.

Institute for Learning. 2006. *Response to the White Paper: further education, raising skills, improving life chances*. IfL. http://www.ifl.ac.uk.

James, D., ed. 2004. *Research in practice: experiences, insights and interventions from the project Transforming Learning Cultures in Further Education*. Building Effective Research Series 5. London: Learning and Skills Research Centre.

———. 2006. Managing 'ragged-trouser philanthropy': the part-time staffing dilemma in the learning and skills sector. Research report ref: 052298. London: LSDA.

Jameson, J., and Y. Hillier. 2003. *Researching post-compulsory education*. London: Continuum International Books Ltd.

Jameson, J., Y. Hillier, and D. Betts. 2004. The ragged-trousered philanthropy of LSC part-time staff. Paper presented at the British Educational Research Association Annual Conference, September 16–18, in Manchester, UK.

Jameson, J., and I. McNay. 2007. *The ultimate FE leadership and management handbook.* London: Continuum.

Kerfoot, D., and S. Whitehead. 1998. 'Boys own' stuff: masculinity and the management of further education. *Sociological Review* 46: 436–457.

Lave, J., and E. Wenger. 1991. *Situated learning: legitimate peripheral participation.* Cambridge, UK: Cambridge University Press

———. 2002. Legitimate peripheral participation in communities of practice. In *Supporting lifelong learning vol 1: perspectives on learning,* ed. R. Harrison, F. Reeve, A. Hanson, and J. Clarke, 11–126. London: Routledge Falmer.

LSC. 2005a. *A clear direction: The Learning and Skills Council's annual report and accounts for 2004/05.* Coventry, UK: Learning and Skills Council. www.lsc.gov.uk/AnnualReport2005/pdf/LSC_Full_report.pdf.

———. 2005b. *LSC annual report and accounts 2004/05.* Coventry, UK: Learning and Skills Council. www.lsc.gov.uk/AnnualReport2005/pdf/LSC_What_weve_been_doing.pdf.

———. 2005c. *Review of further education colleges' financial plans 2005–08 benchmarking further education colleges.* Coventry, UK: Learning and Skills Council. http://readingroom.lsc.gov.uk/Lsc/2005/funding/providers/review-of-fe-colleges-financial-plans-2005-08.pdf.

LSDA. 2005. *'Foster' review.* LSDA Policy Briefing Paper 39. London: Learning and Skills Development Agency.

NATFHE. 2001. *In from the cold? Part-time teaching, professional development and the ILT.* A report of the Union Learning Fund Project led by NATFHE. London: NATFHE.

———. 2005. *Your rights if you work part-time in further education.* Advisory article on part-time working in further education. www.natfhe.org.uk/?id=parttime. (accessed February 6, 2007).

NIACE. 2005. *Eight in ten: adult learners in further education. The report of the independent Committee of Enquiry invited by NIACE to review the state of adult learning in colleges of further education in England.* Leicester, UK: NIACE. http://www.niace.org.uk/Publications/E/eightinten.asp.

Ollin, R. 2005. Professionals, poachers or street-level bureaucrats: government policy, teaching identities and constructive subversions. In *Discourses of Education in the Age of Imperialism,* ed. Jerome Satterthwaite and Elizabeth Atkinson Part 2, Chapter 9, 151–162. Stoke on Trent, UK: Trentham.

Randle, K., and N. Brady. 1997. Further education and the new managerialism. *Journal of Further and Higher Education* 21: 229–238.

Robson, J. 1998. A profession in crisis: status, culture and identity in the further education college. *Journal of Vocational Education and Training* 50, no. 4: 585–607.

———. 2006. *Teacher professionalism in further and higher education: challenges to culture and practice.* London: Routledge

Shain, F. 1999. Managing to lead: women managers in the further education sector. Paper presented at the BERA Annual Conference, September 2–5, in Brighton, UK.

———. 2000. Managing to lead: women managers in the further education sector. *Journal of Further and Higher Education* 24, no. 2: 218–230.

Shain, F., and D. Gleeson. 1999. Under new management: changing conceptions of teacher professionalism and policy in the further education sector. *Journal of Educational Policy* 14: 445–462.

Spenceley, L. 2006. 'Smoke and mirrors': an examination of the concept of professionalism within the FE sector. *Research in Post-Compulsory Education* 11, no. 3: 289–302.

Strauss, A.L., and J. Corbin. 1990. *Basics of qualitative research: grounded theory procedures and techniques.* Newbury Park, CA: Sage.

TLRP. 2005. Improving learning in further education: A new, cultural approach. *Teaching and Learning Research Briefing 12: TLRP ESRC Research Programmes.* www.tlrp.org/pub/documents/HodkinsonRBFinal.pdf.

Expansive and restrictive approaches to professionalism in FE colleges: the observation of teaching and learning as a case in point

Matt O'Leary

What it means to be a 'professional' in further education (FE) in England has been the subject of ongoing debate over the last two decades. In an attempt to codify professionalism, New Labour developed a package of reforms, crystallised by the introduction of professional standards and qualifications and a new inspection framework under Ofsted. These reforms reflected a political desire to improve FE teachers' professional skills and knowledge and prioritised teaching and learning as the main driver for 'continuous improvement'. The observation of teaching and learning (OTL) subsequently emerged as a pivotal tool with which to evaluate and measure improvement, whilst also promoting teacher learning and development. Drawing on recent research into the use of OTL, this paper focuses on two case-study colleges in the West Midlands, whose contrasting OTL practices serve to exemplify expansive and restrictive approaches to professionalism in FE.

Introduction

In recent years, the observation of teaching and learning (OTL) has emerged as an important initiative in the quest for continuous improvement in further education (FE) colleges in England (O'Leary 2011, 2013). Its dominance as the key means of collecting evidence about what goes on in classrooms, underpinned by the aim of improving the quality of teacher knowledge, competence and performance, has been repeatedly endorsed by the custodians of quality for the sector (e.g. Ofsted 2008).

The use of OTL in FE has a relatively short history. It is only over the last two decades that it has become an established practice in colleges, yet in this short space of time it has come to represent the bedrock of quality systems for teaching and learning (O'Leary 2012). Its emergence as a key initiative in the drive for continuous improvement occurred as part of a wider neo-liberal reform agenda to introduce managerialist systems of management in to the public sector on the premise that they would lead to enhanced levels of performance, productivity and accountability (O'Leary 2011). *Managerialism* is a ubiquitous term found in much of the cognate literature on FE and has become associated with how colleges have operated since the early 1990s as others have discussed (e.g. Avis 2003; Ball 2003; Randle and Brady 1997). Whilst it is not my intention to rehearse previous discussions concerning managerialism in any depth in this paper, it is important to acknowledge its link to the emergence of OTL in FE.

A key principle of managerialism was the view that workers could no longer be trusted to do their jobs efficiently and effectively (Robson 1998). This led to the introduction of audit systems and mechanisms of accountability and 'performativity' to monitor output and performance (Ball 2003). The measurement of teachers' performance and productivity was a key part of this new culture and it was in light of this that OTL emerged as an important means of gathering evidence for colleges' quality systems and preparing for Ofsted inspections (O'Leary 2013). The introduction of professional standards and qualifications for teachers in the sector (FENTO 1999; LLUK 2006), along with the formation of a new inspection framework under Ofsted, were key milestones in crystallising increased reliance on OTL as one of the dominant methods with which to gauge improvement and to judge performance.

This paper examines the role that observation plays in shaping notions of professionalism among staff working in two different colleges. The first section of the paper outlines the study's research focus and methodology. The second section, the core of the paper, presents the study's findings and discussion through the narratives of interviewees from two case study colleges. References to relevant literature are embedded throughout and drawn upon when appropriate, as the intention is to use the limited space available to present the narratives of practitioners working in the sector rather than rehearse the plethora of literature on professionalism and professional identity in FE.

The study

The research data that this paper draws on formed part of a wider mixed-methods study using quantitative and qualitative methods of inquiry with a sample of 500 FE staff working in 10 colleges situated across the West Midlands region of England (O'Leary 2011). The study's focus was concerned with investigating the ways in which the professional identity, learning and development of FE tutors were being shaped through the use of OTL. Given the enormity of the data generated and that some are discussed elsewhere (e.g. O'Leary 2013), the scope of this paper is therefore restricted to examining qualitative data from the semi-structured interviews of participants from two of the three case study colleges involved in the second phase of data collection (interviews).

One of the underpinning aims of choosing to explore OTL through a case study approach in the selected colleges was to provide a more richly contextualised response to what Yin (2009) calls the 'how' and 'why' questions of research. Simons (2009) and Yin (2009) contend that one of the strengths of case study research is that it allows a contemporary phenomenon to be examined in depth and 'in the precise socio-political contexts in which programmes and policies are enacted' (Simons 2009, 23). Thus, the term 'case' is used here to refer to context-specific examples of OTL rather than to describe the intensive study of a single institution.

The two 'case study' colleges presented here, referred to henceforth by the pseudonyms 'Middle England' and 'Millennium', were chosen because they provided rich, contrasting examples of the differing contexts, cultures and practices associated with expansive and restrictive approaches to OTL.

In drawing on Engeström's (1994, 2001) notion of 'expansive learning', Fuller and Unwin (2003, 410), in their case studies of UK modern apprenticeships, developed the terms 'expansive' and 'restrictive' as categories of juxtapositional analysis to make sense of, 'the ways in which modern apprentices experience[d] apprenticeship and the opportunities and barriers to learning that the programme produced'. They argued that an apprenticeship that displayed features associated with expansive learning was likely to lead to a, 'stronger and richer learning environment than that comprising features associated with the restrictive end of the continuum' (411–412). They found that expansive approaches typically resulted in more substantive learning opportunities, with apprentices encouraged to reflect more widely on what they were learning. In contrast, restrictive approaches were symptomatic of a technicist interpretation of learning, where apprenticeship was seen as a means to an end, with limited opportunity to access learning and a desire to complete the 'journey' as quickly as possible.

The application of these two juxtapositional terms provided a useful framework for describing and illuminating the study's data and to understand the relationship between the institutional context and practitioners' conceptualisations of professionalism. Thus, the terms 'expansive' and 'restrictive' are used consistently throughout this paper to refer to 'opportunities and barriers to learning', respectively.

Through the narratives of the three participant groups involved in the OTL process, that is, senior managers, observers and observees, the experiences of staff in Middle England College and Millennium College are examined in detail. Each case starts with a brief overview of the college's context and location, which is then followed by three illuminative vignettes from each participant perspective.

Case study 1: Middle England College

Middle England was a medium-sized college situated in a small city in the centre of England. Unlike some of the other urban colleges included in the study, its catchment area was not subject to the typical socio-economic difficulties associated with inner-city areas. Ryan, a tutor and University and Colleges' Union (UCU) representative at the College, encapsulated its profile:

> White, middle-class college and we don't have any of the inner-city problems. I've been here 20 years and I'm still working with people who taught me! The turnover is very slow. I've only ever had three Principals in my time here … it's a kind of *easy* college that hasn't got the tensions, it hasn't got the problems.

Ryan's description of Middle England as an 'easy college' depicted a stable learning culture. His interpretation was confirmed by Paula, the Vice Principal, who referred to the 'soft and gentle approach to life' that she associated with the 'Middle England *way*'.

The senior manager perspective

Paula had been in post as Vice Principal for teaching and learning for seven years. She commented that her main remit was to transform the College's quality systems for teaching and learning. Observation of teaching and learning was, in her words, the 'bedrock' of these systems:

> I was brought in as a Vice Principal to do something about lesson observation and improve it. There were no managers doing the observations when I arrived, it was the staff development officer and a team of people who she got together, who were advanced practitioners in the main. They didn't observe in their own subject area, in fact they deliberately observed outside of their subject area and that led to this sort of contretemps between the managers who were heads of department, but they didn't know what was going on in any of the observation practices.

The picture Paula painted of the previous OTL regime was one of disjuncture. She referred to the 'contretemps between the managers' as they were excluded from the OTL process, yet paradoxically, as she later went on to say, it was their responsibility to ensure and improve the quality of provision in their respective curriculum areas. Paula was sceptical of the previous scheme's effectiveness in addressing the developmental needs of tutors and its role in the quality improvement (QI) cycle. She was critical that it 'wasn't tied in to the formal coaching and development' of tutors and felt that it had become a perfunctory exercise as there was no evidence of any follow-up action after OTL had been carried out, apart from what she referred to as a 'cursory recognition' during their annual appraisal.

One of the first changes she implemented as part of the new approach was to ensure that the remit for OTL was taken away from the central staff development team and control was passed directly to heads and deputy heads of faculty for them to observe tutors in their own curriculum areas. Paula saw this as fundamental to the success of the QI cycle.

As well as changes to its approach to OTL, Paula was keen to emphasise the role of another key development in the learning cultures of the College, which was the introduction of 'Study Centres'. According to Paula, in order to understand the teaching and learning culture of Middle England fully and its efforts to engender a learner-centred focus to its curriculum, it was important to understand the culture of 'Study Centres':

> The other movement of the College which has moved us from a culture of teaching to learning is the Study Centres. It's a curriculum-based area with all of the human and physical resources that students need in that curriculum area, open plan with no walls or as few walls as possible to keep the building up and therefore teaching sessions and drop-in sessions were there for everybody ... We're now into the fifth or sixth year of these and the thing is you can't do didactic teaching in a Study Centre because you're surrounded by six classes going on at once. So you've got to do personalised learning and task-based learning.

Paula saw the Study Centres as instrumental in encouraging tutors to switch from a traditional, teacher-centred approach to one that had a more personalised, learner-centred focus. One of their unforeseen consequences was that they had also led to tutors becoming more accustomed to being observed by their peers, albeit informally. In some cases, this appeared to have helped to break down barriers, tensions and concerns traditionally associated with OTL as a form of surveillance, discussed elsewhere (e.g. O'Leary 2013). Instead of feeling guarded, working alongside colleagues in these Study Centres seemed to trigger a greater sharing of professional knowledge, skills and resources according to Paula:

> What it means is if I'm watching you doing a lesson over there while I'm doing a lesson over here and you're doing something I'd like to know about, I can say 'how did you do that?' And they might say, 'Oh, I went to someone's Passport session and saw them doing it.' And there's much more sharing.

The 'Passport session' that Paula referred to was part of Middle England's staff development programme 'Passport to Success', an online continuous professional development (CPD) booking and tracking system that was accessible to all staff, much of the content of which had evolved from their OTL scheme. Tutors were encouraged to enrol for sessions based on the 'coaching and development' interview with their manager, following their observation. The coaching and development interview had replaced the annual appraisal meeting between line manager and tutor at Middle England. In practice what this meant was that many observers conflated the interview with the post-OTL feedback so that the CPD needs of staff were discussed in conjunction with their observed lesson. For Paula, this change had helped to 'join up' the various stages of the QI cycle in a way that she felt was missing under the previous regime. It had also enabled the senior management to create a transparent audit trail through which to track the CPD journeys of staff across the College.

Paula argued that these two developments (i.e., changes to the OTL approach and the introduction of Study Centres) had been key in helping to transform the learning cultures of the College. She claimed that they had been responsible for increased levels of collaboration between colleagues and the fostering of a collegial trust between observers and observees:

> The way it's helped with teachers is we've got people saying 'don't come and observe that lesson, come and see this one because I'm really struggling with this one and I want you to come and help me' and so it's changing the focus.

Paula's description of the nature of the observer–observee relationship revealed evidence of the openness and collaborative commitment regarded as vital ingredients for meaningful QI and professional development through OTL to occur. There are parallels to recent research in the field of mentoring in FE vis-à-vis the mentor–mentee relationship and what factors are considered to underpin the success of such relationships (Tedder and Lawy 2009). Paula's comments also accentuated the trust between colleagues and resonated with Avis' (2007, 93) conceptualisation of the conditions required for developing expansive notions of professionalism.

As a result of the College's approach to formal OTL, tutors were given a greater sense of ownership and autonomy in deciding the focus and negotiating which sessions they wished to be observed. Although tutors were informed by their line managers towards the start of the academic year in which week their OTL would occur, the observed session was negotiated between the two. This negotiated approach connects with Freire's (2005) assertion of the importance of democratic relations in professional learning, underpinned by collaborative and egalitarian principles.

The OTL process at Middle England seemed to be driven by individual rather than institutional needs, or what Trorey (2002, 2) referred to as 'professional development' (i.e., individual) as opposed to 'staff development' (i.e., institutional). Yet the institution appeared to benefit as well as the individual as there was a continuous 'giving back' to the College community of practice through the Passport to

Success programme and the 'sharing of practice' that Paula referred to above through other outlets, such as the online repository, nicknamed 'Mr Cute', which was created and managed by tutors:

> It's basically a repository but they call it 'Mr Cute' and people are putting things into it all the time and it's part of this whole movement that has come out of observations.

There was a synergy to the strategy adopted by Middle England's SMT to transform the learning cultures of staff and students, exemplified by their approach to OTL and its role in the QI cycle. When asked why she felt their approach had been a success, Paula replied:

> It's about getting them on board, getting them to understand the process and giving them a sense of ownership ... it's used as learning for all of us rather than a judgement.

Paula's response epitomised some of the features of an expansive notion of professionalism – that is, ownership and collective learning (Fuller and Unwin 2003).

The observer perspective

Irene had worked at Middle England for over 15 years in the delivery of NVQs and assessor training. As a curriculum manager, she was involved in observing staff across a broad range of vocational areas in the college formal OTL scheme and in her role as an internal verifier for external awarding bodies whose accredited programmes were taught at the College.

What emerged as an area of contention across several colleges involved in the study was whether observers carried out OTL in their own curriculum areas or were assigned to others. In the following excerpt, Irene argued for the importance of the subject knowledge of the observer:

> When we had the cross-college observation team one of my concerns was that you could be faced with an observer with no idea of your curriculum area. When we had the transition from the team into departments, what we did there was invite a curriculum expert to come along with you as long as the observee agreed, and I did that and I accompanied somebody who did this. Although I didn't do the observation, I certainly gave my input and the good points and the bad points of the session and I think that should be an option for all. Whatever the observation system is, I think the observee should have the right to ask for an expert to be around.

Irene's comments reinforced Paula's earlier account that under the previous system the allocation of observers was random and this was an issue of concern for her. She went on to argue how Middle England's change to a system whereby managers observed within their own faculties had helped to remove some of the anxiety surrounding OTL experienced under the previous regime and helped to establish trust and confidence among staff:

> I think one of the main contributors has been that they got rid of the observation team. They were a bit like the 'police' really! Even though they were teachers, they were still the 'police' coming round to observe you. Then they put it into the faculties and it became your colleagues and I think that's done away with a lot of the anxiety because if you walk around the offices here, you'll have teams of people sitting there and the

programme managers are in with the general teaching staff and there isn't this elitism and the 'police' have gone ... so I would say that the transition from a specific team to bringing it down into your own team level is a big step forwards.

Irene's reference to the previous observation team as the 'police' was a telling remark about the culture surrounding OTL during that era and exemplified the 'punitive' face of teacher assessment referred to by Freire (2005). Her interpretation of the disjuncture between observers and observees resonated with Paula's earlier comments and contrasted noticeably with the subsequent scheme, which seemed to adopt a more transparent, collaborative approach.

Irene's interpretation appeared to vindicate Paula's decision to devolve power to curriculum managers in order to allow them to play an active part in the quality cycle. What came across very strongly in her comments was how important OTL was to her as a means of ascertaining the skills and knowledge base of her team and identifying those areas of practice where additional 'training' needed to be put into place. Irene used OTL as a springboard for engaging in professional dialogue with the members of her team rather than as an end in itself (Peel 2005). The hierarchical divide between observer and observee seemed less marked than under the previous scheme as the two participated in an ongoing process of negotiation and collaboration as part of a collective quest for continuous improvement.

Irene's attitude to those tutors who were assessed as 'requires improvement' or 'inadequate' seemed largely supportive and reflected a commitment to helping them to improve. The way that she carried out her role was what Tilstone (1998) labelled 'partnership observation' (6), but also consistent with Middle England's written policy document on OTL, which stated that:

> Improving the quality of teaching and learning is a *shared* responsibility. This involves Heads of Department and/or Programme Managers working together with teachers to ensure that objectives are discussed and agreed.

The observee perspective

Ryan had taught for over 20 years at Middle England. He was also the Chair of UCU and its main representative in the College. Below, he recounts an anecdote about the previous OTL scheme based on his experience as an observee:

> There were concerns about the scheme. The main concern was that in many areas people were saying that the people doing the observations were not technically qualified. So I was doing something on local government finance and you don't get anything more arcane than local government finance and the observer came in. She was a well-known character in the College, so she was doing her inspection, so she got involved with all the students and all that but I could have been talking complete rubbish about local government finance for all she knew because she didn't have a clue. To be honest it didn't worry me but that was a continuing criticism that had gone on about the old scheme, it did cause a lot of resentment.

Ryan's critique of the previous scheme triangulated with the views of Paula and Irene. His use of the word 'resentment' also highlighted the strength of emotions among staff, reinforcing the negative attitudes towards it, as too did his description of OTL as 'inspection', suggesting that it was seen as a form of 'policing' practice (Gleeson, Davies, and Wheeler 2005).

Talking from a union perspective, Ryan acknowledged the 'new approach' to OTL as positive with a clear focus on the professional development of tutors:

> I think the message we got from the management with the new approach was the new observation scheme was intended to be developmental. It's meant to observe lessons but in the spirit of, 'Well, how does this fit in with your coaching and development?' Now as union officials we were quite pleased with that, you'd be mad not to agree with that. ... My feeling is that actually the system is reasonably open. And secondly as I say, I haven't had any member coming to my door and complain. The system we have now is that programme area managers do the lesson observations and that's an important step forward we think. You know them so they're not being parachuted in and there is an argument that they are much closer to your area of work.

Much of Ryan's description of the OTL scheme and the union's reaction to it echoed the original rationale put forward by Paula. Unlike the scheme it had replaced, there was evidence of a shared, transparent understanding across the College of what its aims were and staff working towards a shared goal. Besides, the fact that Ryan mentioned that he had not received a single complaint about it in all his time as a union representative was not only noteworthy in itself, but especially bearing in mind how it has 'become an increasingly common flash point in colleges, triggering local negotiations, and in some places industrial disputes' in recent times (UCU 2009, 1).

Case study 2: context and location of Millennium College

Millennium College was situated in rural settings in the centre of England. During the first phase of the study it was a small institution with fewer than two thousand students enrolled, specialising in land-based programmes. A team of just three observers were responsible for OTL across the College. However, by phase two it had completed a merger with two other local colleges and had become the smallest of four campuses of a new, much larger college with a capacity for 20,000 full- and part-time students.

The senior manager perspective

At the time of interview Graham had been in post as Director of Quality at Millennium for less than a year. He had held a similar post at one of the other two colleges prior to the merger for several years, before which he had worked in management in the automotive and engineering industries.

In contrast to Middle England's approach to OTL, Graham chose to implement a similar model to the one that had been in place when Paula was appointed and which she was so eager to remove. In other words, Millennium chose not to allocate managers to observe their own departmental staff but assigned them randomly to different departments:

> Researcher: I'm just thinking about the observers who carry out formal observations. Who do they observe? Are they doing it cross college?
>
> Graham: Well, they never do their own staff.
>
> Researcher: Oh right, is that a deliberate strategy?

Graham: Absolutely! Managers are very competitive people! And part of the monthly report I produce for the Executive has the breakdown by faculty area and I know it's a competitive world when it comes to management.

Researcher: So does this mean then that the people that get allocated to observe is a completely random selection of people?

Graham: Yes, totally random.

Graham's comment about managers being 'very competitive people' depicted a very different conceptualisation of working cultures at Millennium to the one described by Paula at Middle England. Instead of fostering a community of collaboration and cooperation between colleagues, Millennium's approach seemed to reflect a managerialist model that insisted on regular surveillance coupled with performative measures.

Although Graham was not explicit in his use of the word *trust*, it could be inferred that the decision not to allow managers to observe tutors in their own department was fuelled by a lack of trust in their integrity to assess them without bias on account of their 'competitive' nature. Nevertheless, it is important to acknowledge that an *inter*-departmental rather than an *intra*-departmental model of OTL is not uncommon in colleges as it is argued that it minimises observer bias in the assessment process. A similar rationale underpins the decision of some colleges to employ external consultants to carry out OTL on an annual basis.

At a later point during the interview, the issue of trust resurfaced in the context of the College's approach to ungraded OTL carried out by mentors, and it was interesting to note that in this instance Graham revealed a very different conceptualisation of the observer–observee relationship:

Researcher: The people that are coaches or mentors and carry out peer observations, are they a completely separate group to the observers that carry out the formal observations?

Graham: Oh, yes! I've kept that separation and would protect it with my life! Mentors need to be trusted so there is no point where they would say 'that was a grade four'.

There was a curious contrast to how Graham viewed the two contexts/models of OTL, which illustrated some of the paradoxes and tensions associated with the Millennium approach. On the one hand, he insinuated that managers were too competitive to be trusted to observe their own staff as part of the graded OTL scheme and thus were deliberately prevented from contributing to that part of the QI cycle. On the other hand, he acknowledged the importance of trust in establishing a positive relationship between mentors and the tutors to whom they were assigned when carrying out peer OTL.

Graham further revealed how the allocation of mentors was seen as a punitive measure as it only occurred in the event of a grade three or four, thus the notion of trust seemed tainted from the outset and was further compromised by the pressure on the observee and mentor to raise the level of performance by at least one grade within a six-week period:

> Our policy is that every teacher will be observed twice in the academic year. The second observation is waived if the teacher achieves a grade one or grade two in the first observation, so you get your one or two and you're done for the year, you can breathe a sigh of relief. The big tension is with the threes because the three gets you, 'Oh no, not one of those mentors!' They get a grade three and they get allocated a mentor so it's almost like the mentor has become the punishment and this worries me.

Following Ofsted's proclamation that 'satisfactory is not good enough' any more (Ofsted 2008, 4) and the subsequent re-branding of a grade three from 'satisfactory' to 'requires improvement', the response of Millennium and other colleges has been to assign mentors to work with those tutors awarded a grade three or four in order to help them to raise their level of performance and consequently improve the overall college grade profile.

Graham's comments above indicated that the allocation of a mentor was seen as a punitive consequence rather than as an opportunity to further develop one's professional practice. This was hardly surprising given the 'high stakes' nature (Boardman and Woodruff 2004) of graded OTL and the subsequent pressure for tutors awarded a grade three or four to 'up their performance' (Graham) within a short timescale.

It was difficult to pinpoint the underlying principles behind Millennium's approach to OTL and whether the merger had contributed to creating what seemed a contradictory picture, compared to, for example, that of Middle England. Having said that, Graham's comments implied that the role of managers during graded OTL was largely that of judges rather than active collaborators in the coaching and development of tutors. It appeared that the latter was the domain of mentors, and only then in the event of those tutors who were graded as a three or four.

The observer perspective

Abdul, Molly and Cristina were three experienced observers who, prior to the merger, formed part of a close-knit team on one campus, all having worked mainly on ITT and CPD programmes for many years. A common theme in their joint interview was how the merger had revealed differences in working cultures and conflicting approaches to OTL across the new campuses. They referred to differences in approach and beliefs between the different campuses. Their 'approach' to OTL was based on the belief that it was a 'shared partnership', the focus of which was 'developmental' and 'constructive', similar to Tilstone's (1998) notion of 'partnership observation'.

Given their background in ITT and CPD, one might argue that it was understandable that they had a natural 'empathy' with the teachers on their campus. Besides, having worked in such a close-knit team for so long on the smallest of four campuses suggested they might have been in a better position than some of their colleagues from much larger campuses to develop a personalised relationship with their colleagues. Notwithstanding these suppositions, a strong message to come across in interview was that despite the changes resulting from the merger, they were determined not to compromise their professional values and beliefs in their role as observers.

As an example of this Molly talked about how as a team they had always prioritised OTL appointments regardless of other managerial commitments, whereas their fellow observers at other campuses appeared to regard them as less important and would cancel them with little or no notice. All three suggested that the model of OTL in use at Millennium's two main campuses was designed to satisfy systems of performance management and accountability rather than the developmental needs of tutors. Abdul exemplified this in talking about the 'difference in paperwork' and how, under the new systems of Millennium, the forms were 'more prescriptive' and indicative of what he referred to as 'a return to the bad old days of observation forms with four million tick boxes'.

However, rather than abandoning their previous approach they looked for ways to retain its core principles whilst also complying with these new systems and practices, as commented in the following extract:

Abdul: I'm fighting it because regardless of what people above tell me I should be doing, I'm still going to be doing the observations in a supportive way. I can write it up in any way they want but I'm still going to carry out the process in a supportive way.

Researcher: Do you feel any conflict in what you're being asked to do and the way in which you're, to use your words, you're 'fighting it'?

Molly: Shall I answer that for you? I think we do if we're honest. We work so closely as a team with the same philosophy and understandings of what we're trying to achieve and how, and I think if you ask us to define our roles, *support* would have been very high up the list and I think now it's more as Abdul says, it's more about appraisal now. We almost seem to be going back to the days where we're measuring what has been going on rather than improving what can come.

The determination of these observers not to compromise their commitment to maintaining the formative focus of OTL in the face of a wider institutional move towards using it as an accountability mechanism exemplified what Shain and Gleeson (1999) referred to as 'strategic compliance'. By acting as 'strategic compliers', they were able to preserve their pedagogic principles, whilst still fulfilling the requirements of college systems of accountability.

Closely related to the notion of strategic compliance is Wallace and Hoyle's (2005) term, 'principled infidelity'. For these observers, principled infidelity was a way of managing the tensions between policy and practice and the pressures of managerialism in a newly formed college. Their comments revealed a conflict between their professional values and the expectations and requirements of the managerialist college systems. What was clear from their comments was that they found themselves having to adjust to what Abdul referred to as an 'intense level of micro-management' that they had not been used to, which suggested they were able to operate with more autonomy under the previous systems and in high-trust working contexts (Avis 2003).

Cristina talked about how the new systems had 'put things into silos' with regard to roles and responsibilities. Abdul provides an example of this in the following extract:

Abdul: In terms of observation, we were told just last weekend that as mentors we would now not be on the observation team so they now very much see the two roles as being completely different.

Researcher: Do you want to expand on what you mean by that as in what 'they' see as different?

Abdul: That the college management now see that if you are having a coaching or mentoring role then you should not be on the formal observation team.

One of the consequences of 'put[ting] things into silos', as Cristina stated, was that it made it more difficult to achieve the 'joined up thinking' between elements of the QI cycle that Paula referred to above, as opportunities for working collaboratively and sharing practice across the College were reduced. Abdul's comments also linked into Graham's conceptualisation of the observer–observee relationship, discussed above. What these two models of OTL revealed was a clear delineation in power and authority where the responsibility for judgement was preserved for senior managers and the 'repair work', alluded to by Abdul below, became the mentor's responsibility:

I think what unnerves me is that you've got a grade four and you will be observed within six weeks so there is a reliance there on the fact that you can turn someone around in six weeks and, if not, well fair enough, we don't care and we're going to take you down the incompetency route.

Abdul's use of the term to 'turn someone around in six weeks' provided an insight into the way in which the senior management of Millennium perceived the mentor's role. It was almost as if the mentor was required to take on the mantle of *repair technician* as s/he was tasked with repairing the *faulty goods* and re-circulating them into the system once they had passed the approved *safety standards*. As Abdul pointed out, unless the observee was able to improve their grade in the follow-up OTL six weeks later, they were likely to be faced with disciplinary procedures. Interestingly, in the case of Millennium, graded OTL seemed to operate largely on a punitive basis as not only were tutors faced with the threat of disciplinary procedures, but also the loss of their annual salary increment. Thus graded OTL was being used as a form of performance-related pay.

Finally, another area of OTL practice that the three observers were keen to discuss was the disclosure of grades and how prior to the merger they had trialled a model in which grades were removed from the assessment:

Abdul: We did try to disassociate formal observations from appraisal in terms of trying to make all of our formal observations more formative and we managed to get the lesson observation grade taken off the appraisal form for a while. So, clearly, we have now moved completely away from that again and everything is performance driven and that's where I think that's where we made all of our advances in improving the quality of teaching by getting people on side, being formative as opposed to punitive.

Researcher: What was the rationale behind that move away from the previous system?

Abdul: We started to not give numerical grades for observations as we felt people concentrated on the number not the feedback and we felt that that worked really well but then the Principal decided one day that Ofsted wouldn't like that and everything came to a halt so we're obviously back with numerical grades now.

Molly: Yes and we did it for just under a year and the impact was quite startling. The quality of learning that was going on rose because staff listened to the developmental feedback rather than focusing on 'oh I've got a three'. We had got staff on side with observations and they were no longer terrorised of having someone in the classroom. They became far more accepting.

Their account gave the impression that removing the grade from the OTL process was liberating and helped to break down some of the negative barriers (i.e., anxiety, suspicion, etc.) associated with graded OTL. It enabled them as observers to gain the trust of tutors and to engage in meaningful, collaborative work, which subsequently led to improvements in the quality of teaching. By concentrating on the feedback and not the grade, the formative aspect of the OTL process took on a greater significance and tutors were more disposed to engaging in professional dialogue about their practice.

The observee perspective

Donna, Anne and Gavin were tutors with varying periods of service at Millennium. Donna and Anne were both employed as full-time tutors of basic skills, whereas Gavin, a full-time farmer, taught agricultural studies on a part-time basis. Although they were interviewed separately (Donna and Anne in a paired interview and Gavin individually), common themes emerged in their responses. For example, all three manifested a sense of unease and frustration regarding some of the changes that had occurred as a result of the merger. Gavin seemed less concerned than Donna and Anne, as he stressed that his livelihood did not depend on his teaching at the College.

Donna and Anne talked about how the working cultures and ethos of what was, in their words, a 'positive', 'close-knit' college had been affected by the merger. They talked about experiencing a changeover to a more 'business-like', performative approach to OTL and recounted the decision of management to publish the names of staff whose lessons were graded as a one during the last round of formal OTL across the College as an example:

Donna: There was an outbreak of emails congratulating people on getting grade ones which I thought was bad, very unsupportive from the management team.

Researcher: Just to individuals?

Donna: No! It was an all staff email thanking them 'blah, blah, blah' with congratulations and 'you too can aspire to be like' …

Researcher: So those individuals who got grade ones were named?

Donna: Yes! Well the people who got the grade ones were mainly embarrassed to be named and they didn't want people to know so straight away they took away their right to confidentiality by publishing their names, although thinking about it there were also a few who were walking round as if they were the 'bee's knees' and no surprise that they're the ones who are crap teachers anyway. People who didn't get a grade one, like myself, then felt somehow inferior to these people. It made me question whether or not I'm up to the job … if you don't see your name in this

> space the inference is that you're not as good as them, which isn't good really because it's kind of divisive for a whole team and if you've got members in your own team then it makes them feel uncomfortable.

Donna argued that the 'divisive' repercussions of disclosing grades could be felt on both an individual and collective level, and such practice was therefore seen to militate against the fostering of cooperative working relationships between tutors. Besides, in confirming the views of the observers discussed previously, Donna went on to describe how OTL was 'something that is done to you' and hence a less supportive experience for tutors under the new regime, as the extract below reveals. There was a distinct lack of collaboration and ownership of the OTL process in the way Donna described her recent experience as an observee and little evidence of how it linked up to tutors' wider CPD. Similarly, Gavin talked about how the feedback had become 'less supportive now' than in previous years. The two responses below highlighted some of the tensions surrounding the use of OTL at Millennium:

Researcher: How would you describe your colleagues' attitudes towards observation?

Donna: I don't know anybody who is happy about them. They're all pretty much the same about them when they know they're coming … just glad to get it over and done with I think.

Gavin: It does highlight the weak areas but it's just how they're dealt with that's the main problem and the fact that certainly here you feel like you're under threat when you have your observation; it's quite an upsetting time to be fair.

At the end of both interviews all three observees were asked if they had any ideas as to how OTL might be made more beneficial to them and their colleagues. They all emphasised the importance of it being conducted as a 'supportive' process, once again reinforcing the values of the previous team of observers.

Conclusion

This paper has discussed contrasting approaches to professionalism and professional learning through the use of OTL in two colleges, Middle England and Millennium. Each college's approach to OTL has been examined through the narratives of three groups of participants. Table 1 categorises the key features associated with the differing approaches to OTL in evidence in these two colleges according to a 'restrictive–expansive continuum'.

The way in which staff experienced and engaged with OTL in these two colleges seemed to be heavily influenced by the learning cultures of the college itself. The commitment of the college SMT to promote particular notions of professionalism was crucial in establishing an institutional ethos towards OTL, which was cascaded, both implicitly and explicitly, to observers and observees.

Restrictive approaches to OTL displayed a clear delineation of power as to who controlled the agenda and the production of data, which was based on hierarchical seniority. Whereas in expansive approaches, the power differential between observer and observee was less hierarchically marked and seemed to embrace a more

Table 1. Restrictive–expansive continuum of approaches to OTL.

Restrictive approaches to OTL	Expansive approaches to OTL
• Emphasis on *measuring* teaching and learning by allocating individual grades from Ofsted 4-point scale • Emphasis on summative aspects of OTL • Observees have no input in which lesson is observed nor the focus • Random allocation of observers to different subject areas • 'Fetishisation' of the observed lesson – forms crux of judgements about professional competence and capability • OTL is disconnected from other college systems of CPD, often the domain of 'Quality Unit' • Limited opportunity for observee input or ownership in OTL process • Clear delineation of power between observer and observee based on hierarchical seniority • Observer as 'judgement maker' • OTL provokes increased levels of stress and anxiety	• Emphasis on *improving* teaching and learning, often ungraded or grade seen as of minor importance • Emphasis on formative aspects of OTL as part of CPD • Greater autonomy for observees to decide the lesson and focus of OTL • Observer often a specialist in the subject area of the observee • OTL is seen as one means of collecting evidence about classroom practice and teacher performance • Convergence across CPD and QA units of colleges, OTL is part of multiple communities of practice • Balanced distribution of power in which observee's voice is valued • Power differential between observer and observee less hierarchically marked • Observer as supportive mentor • OTL welcomed as an opportunity for reciprocal professional learning

Notes: OTL = observation of teaching and learning, CPD = continuous professional development, QA = quality assurance.

balanced, collaborative distribution of power in which the observee's voice was regarded as valid as the observer's.

The findings from Middle England suggested a broad triangulation of interpretations across all three groups. Overall, OTL was seen as a supportive, formative process based on a desire to promote collaboration among colleagues. These views reflected some of the characteristics associated with expansive notions of professional learning highlighted in the work of Fuller and Unwin (2003). For example, in the context of personal development they identified the importance of 'belonging to multiple communities of practice' (417). Such instances of multiple communities of practice at Middle England were embodied in the 'Passport to Success' scheme, 'Mr Cute' and its Study Centres.

In contrast, restrictive approaches emphasised the summative outcome as the *raison d'être* of OTL, thus leading to a *fetishisation* of the observed lesson. The formative element was often either absent from the OTL process or given very limited treatment. In the case of Millennium, it also tended to be disconnected and dealt with as part of a separate, fragmented exercise in which those tutors who were evaluated as a grade three or four were treated as individual problems. In many ways, such restrictive approaches to OTL encapsulated Freire's (2005) interpretation of the punitive use of teacher evaluation that, 'we evaluate to punish and almost never to improve teachers' practice. In other words, we evaluate to punish and not to educate' (13).

There was a pressure to perform on an individual level, exacerbating the high-stakes nature of the assessment and often militating against the fostering of collaborative, collegial relationships between observer and observee. In such instances, both parties found their roles demarcated and prescribed for them by performance management systems designed primarily to collect auditable evidence, allowing little opportunity to influence the focus or running of the OTL process. Nonetheless, some of the observers' comments at Millennium College exemplified Wallace and Hoyle's (2005) notion of principled infidelity and illustrated their determination to resist the dominant discourses of managerialism and performativity.

So, is it possible to arrive at an integrated model of OTL that meets the demands of performative quality assurance (QA) systems and the CPD needs of its teachers? Or does this require two separate models, each with differing purposes? The findings from this research underline that such integration is not unproblematic. One of the biggest obstacles would appear to be the issue of grading and the importance attached to it. Where restrictive approaches were evident, the reliance on and importance attached to OTL grades as key indicators of professional competence seemed to correlate with low levels of trust and professional autonomy. Yet when the grading element was removed, this appeared to promote improved levels of trust between colleagues and helped to break down some of the negative associations surrounding the use of OTL.

Perhaps then, the answer lies not in seeking to create a dual purpose model in which expansive approaches are integrated into a predominantly performative initiative, but one that prioritises teacher learning above all else. Such a move would undoubtedly go against the grain of current normalised models of graded OTL and signify a bold step in re-defining its use in the sector. Whether or not colleges are prepared to take such a step remains to be seen, but equally, ignoring the distorting and counterproductive consequences of this initiative is surely not an option for policy makers and practitioners alike committed to the ongoing improvement of teaching and learning in FE.

References

Avis, J. 2003. "Re-thinking Trust in a Performative Culture: The Case of Education." *Journal of Education Policy* 18 (3): 315–332.

Avis, J. 2007. *Education, Policy and Social Justice: Learning and Skills.* London: Continuum.

Ball, S. J. 2003. "The Teacher's Soul and the Terrors of Performativity." *Journal of Education Policy* 18 (2): 215–228.

Boardman, A. G., and A. L. Woodruff. 2004. "Teacher Change and 'High-stakes' Assessment: What Happens to Professional Development?" *Teaching and Teacher Education* 20 (6): 545–557.

Engeström, Y. 1994. *Training for Change: New Approach to Instruction and Learning in Working Life*. Geneva: International Labour Office.
Engeström, Y. 2001. "Expansive Learning at Work: Toward an Activity Theoretical Reconceptualization." *Journal of Education and Work* 14 (1): 133–156.
Freire, P. 2005. *Teachers as Cultural Workers – Letters to Those Who Dare Teach*. Cambridge, MA: Westview Press.
Fuller, A., and L. Unwin. 2003. "Learning as Apprentices in the Contemporary UK Workplace: Creating and Managing Expansive and Restrictive Participation." *Journal of Education and Work* 16 (4): 407–426.
Further Education National Training Organisation. 1999. *National Standards for Teaching and Supporting Learning in Further Education in England and Wales*. London: FENTO.
Gleeson, D., J. Davies, and E. Wheeler. 2005. "On the Making and Taking of Professionalism in the Further Education Workplace." *British Journal of Sociology of Education* 26 (4): 445–460.
Lifelong Learning UK. 2006. *New Overarching Professional Standards for Teachers, Tutors and Trainers in the Lifelong Learning Sector*. London: LLUK.
O'Leary, M. 2011. "The Role of Lesson Observation in Shaping Professional Identity, Learning and Development in Further Education Colleges in the West Midlands." Unpublished PhD Thesis, University of Warwick, September.
O'Leary, M. 2012. "Exploring the Role of Lesson Observation in the English Education System: A Review of Methods, Models and Meanings." *Professional Development in Education* 38 (5): 791–810.
O'Leary, M. 2013. "Surveillance, Performativity and Normalised Practice: The Use and Impact of Graded Lesson Observations in Further Education Colleges." *Journal of Further and Higher Education* 37 (5): 694–714.
Ofsted. 2008. *How Colleges Improve*. London: Ofsted Publications Centre.
Peel, D. 2005. "Peer Observation as a Transformatory Tool?" *Teaching in Higher Education* 10 (4): 489–504.
Randle, K., and M. Brady. 1997. "Managerialism and Professionalism in the 'Cinderella Service'." *Journal of Vocational Education and Training* 49 (1): 121–139.
Robson, J. 1998. "A Profession in Crisis: Status, Culture and Identity in the Further Education College." *Journal of Vocational Education and Training* 50 (4): 585–607.
Shain, F., and D. Gleeson. 1999. "Teachers' Work and Professionalism in the Post Incorporated FE Sector." *Education and Social Justice* 1 (3): 55–63.
Simons, H. 2009. *Case Study Research in Practice*. London: Sage.
Tedder, M., and R. Lawy. 2009. "The Pursuit of 'Excellence': Mentoring in Further Education Initial Teacher Training in England." *Journal of Vocational Education & Training* 61 (4): 413–429.
Tilstone, C. 1998. *Observing Teaching and Learning – Principles and Practice*. London: David Fulton.
Trorey, G. 2002. "Introduction: Meeting the Needs of the Individual and the Institution." In *Professional Development and Institutional Needs*, edited by G. Trorey and C. Cullingford, 1–14. Aldershot: Ashgate.
University and College Union. 2009. "Lesson Observation UCU Guidelines." Accessed February 22, 2010. http://www.ucu.org.uk/index.cfm?articleid=2969
Wallace, M., and E. Hoyle. 2005. "Towards Effective Management of a Reformed Teaching Profession." Paper presented at the 4th Seminar of the ESRC Teaching and Learning Research Programme Thematic Seminar Series 'Changing Teacher Roles, Identities and Professionalism', King's College London. Accessed September 22, 2010. http://www.kcl.ac.uk/content/1/c6/01/41/66/paper-wallace.pdf
Yin, R. K. 2009. *Case Study Research: Design and Methods*. 4th ed. London: Sage.

Professionalism: doing a good job!

Denis Feather

This paper considers the concept of professionalism via perceptions (real or imagined) of lecturers delivering higher education business programmes (HEBPs) in further education colleges in England. The study comprised 26 in-depth interviews conducted in the Yorkshire and Humber region in the UK. The study builds on Perkin's views of a professional society, which is then applied to education. The paper will add to existing knowledge by identifying that the term profession is not only complex and subjective, but Janus-faced, which may lead to role conflict. It was not surprising that the interviewees found it difficult to define professionalism; nevertheless, it was found that many did hold to a perceived individual professional code of praxis and/or idea of expected behaviour.

Introduction

The purpose of this paper is to consider the concept of professionalism from a higher education (HE) in further education (FE) perspective (either real or imagined), through the lens of business lecturers delivering higher education business programmes (HEBPs) in further education colleges (FECs) in the north east of England. The study adopted an interpretivist approach, where 26 semi-structured, individual, in-depth interviews were conducted. These narratives offered a valuable insight into how these lecturers perceived their professional status, and that of the 'communities of practice' they worked in. The study highlights that there is some accord between the secondary and primary data, but also identifies that the term 'professionalism' may be used as a managerialist control mechanism, that is, if the lecturers do not comply with requests of management, they may be seen as being obstructive and/or unprofessional. As Friedson (2001, 13) writes: 'The concept of profession tends to keep us from seeing those with that label as workers.' He argues that by using the term professional or professionalism, it sets apart those who see themselves as working in special positions, compared to others who work in other roles, or what Friedson (2001) refers to as the 'humble occupations'.

An overview of professionalism

Professionalism is both a highly complex and subjective term (Feather 2009) to define. This is evidenced by the lack of accord between different authors on what constitutes professional and/or professionalism and therefore it may prove difficult to offer any real clarity (Gleeson, Davies, and Wheeler 2005). The obfuscation is in large part down to different authors using the terms professional and professionalism interchangeably. However, it is accepted that others may see and apply these differently, but acting professionally could be viewed by lecturers in some FECs as being, or aspiring to be seen as a professional. This is evidenced in the work of Perkin (2002) on *The Rise of Professional Society: England Since 1880*. In this text, he offers many variations of the term professional, but in addition, also highlights how professionalism is not only specialised, but also dynamic and ever evolving. He writes:

> The world we have gained and may be about to lose is a consequence of myriad driven activities which have only one thing in common: they are increasingly specialised, increasingly diverse, increasingly skilled – in a word, increasingly professional. (Perkin 2002, 3)

Perkin (2002) goes on to argue that from this increased professionalism within society, professionalism itself has, in his view, become another ruling class 'permeating society from top to bottom' (Perkin 2002, 3). He highlights that professionalism is now a class in addition to those of the working, middle, and upper classes in society (Perkin 2002). A further inference could be that every individual within society could lay claim to being a professional. However, is this reality or merely imagined? The point about every person being able to lay claim to being a professional may have some relevance in that the term 'professional' has become a part of everyday language, and to some extent may be becoming somewhat watered down in the status that Perkin (2002) is suggesting. Meek (1988) quoting Geertz (1973, 4) writes along similar lines when he likens professionalism to a spider's web, that is, 'that man is an animal suspended in webs of significance he himself [*sic*] has spun'. This would fit with the imaginary viewpoint of professionalism and further evidence that people may use professionalism to mean anything they perceive identifies them as being at the top of their field, offering the opportunity for these individuals to be viewed as the guardians of high quality and ethical standards. Furthermore, some webs that people spin may be based on different attitudes, values and beliefs of what constitutes professionalism and subsequently, being a profession. This primarily may be due to the different cultures in which they are raised as children, and the communities of practice they are immersed in when at work (Silver 2003; Simmons 2003; Hofstede and Hofstede 2005; Goodhall 2009; Feather 2011a).

On the subject of knowledge – which Perkin (2002) refers to as specialist, or expert knowledge – Mintzberg (1993) argues that organisations need experts and their knowledge; on this he writes 'the organization has need of specialized knowledge, notably because certain decisions are highly technical ones, [therefore] certain experts attain considerable informal power' (Mintzberg 1993, 109). Mintzberg's (1993) views may also apply in education, as knowledge is a lecturer's core skill.

When considering status between different educational institutions, knowledge may also represent the perceived hierarchical differences (Hall 2002) between higher education (HE) and further education (FE), and now HE in FE (Feather 2011a, 2011b). As such, groups may have power to influence, or even reverse, managerial decisions due to the strength of the communities of practice (Clegg 2008; Nagy and Burch 2009; Feather 2011a; Gale, Turner, and McKenzie 2011), or agency (Archer 2000) that may be found in any organisation and its different departments. Therefore, being part of a community of practice and having agency (power to control certain aspects of one's work through numbers) may enable these groups to negotiate their professional status. On this latter point Mintzberg (1993, 197) writes: 'not only do professionals control their own work, but they also seek collective control of the administrative decisions that affect them'. Archer (2008) appears to be in accord with this view when reflecting on academic authenticity and legitimacy, believing that individuals and groups within departments or institutions may compete to ensure that their specific needs, 'interests, characteristics and identities are accorded recognition and value' (Archer 2008, 386). This becomes ubiquitous when Gale, Turner, and McKenzie (2011) argue that:

> There is an expectation for college lecturers to develop HE practice styles and under-take HE-related activities such as scholarly activity and research in an environment not traditionally associated with these activities. (160)

The problem here, especially in FE, is that lecturers may not have as much control over what they do as they once had. One caveat to remember in relation to communities of practice or agency, as discussed by Meek (1988) and Feather (2011a), is that individuals may have separate itineraries to those of the department or institution, which may or may not be aligned to the policies, procedures, goals and objectives set by management. Nixon (2001) may be in agreement with this view, arguing that the professional society will inevitably, by its very nature, be tainted. That is, he believes it will have an undertow of conflicting tendencies due to managerialism and marketisation (Nixon 2001). Effectively, this will not only impact on society, but on higher education in particular (Nixon 2001). He argues that management and 'the marketisation of university education has led to an increased emphasis on quality control, and to the wholesale auditing of state institutions' (Nixon 2001, 179). Nixon et al. (2001, 231) write that:

> Key questions in the debate concern the extent to which university teachers now constitute: a profession divided against itself; a set of occupations so diverse in their practices that the term 'professional' may no longer be applicable in all or even most cases; a new proletariat with very little opportunity, and even less encouragement, to exercise independent judgement and self regulation; or a new professional grouping based on alternative values and aspirations.

These various issues offer an insight into why Nixon believes the higher education profession is being deprofessionalised (Nixon 2001).

The above is not a new occurrence in education; FE has felt these same effects for some time and has had to deal with not just one governmental quango (in the UK) of quality assurance auditing systems, but two – one for FE, and one for HE in FE (Parry and Thompson 2002). This adds further weight to the view of some lecturers in HE and HE in FE that their role is being deprofessionalised and de-skilled (Shain 1998; Nixon 2001). From this it becomes obvious that the managerial concepts used and applied in the commercial sector do not fit neatly (as UK governments past and present perceive), or can be simply applied to the public sector

(in this case education), and as a result, they appear to be having both a serious and damaging effect on education as a whole (Wolf 2011). Borrowing from Castells (2010, 31) when quoting David Hooson:

> The urge to express one's identity, and to have it recognized tangibly by others, is increasingly contagious and has to be recognized as an elemental force even in the shrunken, apparently homogenizing, high-tech world of the end of the twentieth century.

Obviously Castells (2010) was discussing identity within society as a whole, but I would argue that this viewpoint could be extrapolated to include societies within organisations.

Method

The research methods adopted for this study were from a qualitative perspective, using a mixed philosophical approach of interpretivism and ethnography (Saunders, Lewis, and Thornhill 2007; Teddlie and Tashakkori 2009). The former was because I wished to understand lecturers' perceptions of the terms 'professional' and 'professionalism'. The latter was because I was employed in a FEC delivering HEBPs for nearly two years so I was grounded in the culture and in the ways in which the FEC I worked for practised and delivered HE. To this end, I wished to establish if those lecturers who taught HEBPs in different FECs had similar points of view in relation to professionalism.

In total 26 individual in-depth interviews were conducted within a number of FECs throughout the Yorkshire and Humber region in the UK. The sample of interviewees were selected from those who 'self-identified' via the 96 questionnaires returned out of the 154 sent out to FECs in England. In total 52 lecturers self-identified that they were willing to take further part in the study by agreeing to be interviewed.

Using a purposive sampling approach, I selected a representative sample that incorporated the following factors: gender, years of teaching experience, age, different ethnicities, part- and full-time contracted staff, education qualifications, and geographic distribution. The interviews were approximately 60 minutes in duration and were recorded and later fully transcribed. Content and thematic analysis was then employed to identify themes and/or strings of words that were evident in the narratives (BERA 2003). These were coded using words and titles, for example, 'costs', 'professional', 'customers', 'doing a good job', and 'currency' – this latter code incorporated the string 'keeping up-to-date'. As Denscombe (2012, 281; original emphasis) writes: 'Content analysis can be used with any "text"... *Break*[ing] *the text down into smaller component units*. The unit for analysis can be each and every word.'

Generalisations cannot be made due to the small sample size, but the findings from this study conducted within business schools in FECs may be extrapolated to other FECs and their business schools/departments, and/or other educational departments within those FECs.

I have quoted the interviewees verbatim and have in square brackets made a note of their gesticulations or actions. Additionally, where the respondent has paused for thought, for example four seconds, this will appear as '[*four seconds*]' within the narrative. The lengths of some of these pauses and subsequent gesticulations are as important as the spoken word (Robson 2002) and give the reader a flavour of the personality of the people who offered their narrative to aid understanding of their perceptions.

Written permission was acquired from the principals of the various FECs approached for the study, and informed consent acquired from the interviewees before the interviews and recording commenced. The British Education Research Association (BERA) guidelines were adhered to (BERA 2011). To this end, the identities of the participating institutions and those interviewed as part of this study will remain anonymous, and their individual rights preserved. Subsequently, the identities of the individuals that appear in this study are expressed as 'Int. 1', and no individual FEC is referred to.

Discussion

As highlighted in the review of the literature, the idiom of professionalism is both a complex and highly subjective term to define. There are too many works to list or cover here, but this subject is addressed by leading authors from a range of different perspectives (see Farrugia 1996; Bayer and Braxton 1998; Clow 2001; Friedson 2001; Nixon 2001; Perkin 2002; Bathmaker and Avis 2005a; Beck and Young 2005; Gleeson, Davies, and Wheeler 2005; Archer 2008; Turner, McKenzie, and Stone 2009; Gale, Turner, and McKenzie 2011).

Having said this, some of the above works have been considered and discussed with a view to offering a flavour of current thinking about the term professionalism. When defining professionalism, Schuck, Gordon, and Buchanan (2008, 540) write as follows: 'Professionalism is commonly understood as an individual's adherence to a set of standards, code of conduct or collection of qualities that characterise accepted practice within a particular area of activity.' Farrugia (1996) wrote along similar lines, but suggested that professionalism was an indication of a person's beliefs which are based on the person's knowledge, experiences and values. Professionalism 'implies openness and exposure to scrutiny whereby one's pronouncements, beliefs, values and actions can be analysed and evaluated for their validity' (Farrugia 1996, 1). Interviewee (Int.) 8 spoke along similar lines to that of Farrugia (1996) and Schuck, Gordon, and Buchanan (2008), when asked to define the term professionalism. He stated:

Oh my God! [*shouting*]. Right, it's err [*eight seconds*] it's a code of behaviour [*seven seconds*] and that the behaviours displayed can either be classed as being professional or not [*five seconds*] and I know your next question is 'What sort of behaviours are you talking about here?' I think behaviours from our point of view are behaviours in relation to how we relate to students. The currency of the material we present to them, the erm [*four seconds*] equality of assessment opportunities that we provide people. The integrity and honesty that we have with our students and with each other [*six seconds*]. All those things I define as being professional.

Int. 22 believed the terms 'professional' and 'professionalism' are now used in different contexts, and for different reasons, which is in accord with Perkin's (2002) views discussed earlier in the paper. When defining how she perceives a professional, Int. 22 says the following:

> Oh, I think that's very difficult [*starts laughing*], erm, because as you say ... everybody does talk about being professional, and so on. Doing the job to their best ability [*four seconds*], erm [*seven seconds*] that just sounds a bit crass [*laughs loudly*]. Erm [*eight seconds*] I don't think [*seven seconds*] I know some people say being professional means holding a professional qualification. I don't think the word is used like that anymore. People tend to use it now about being professional in what they do, as in giving a good service, doing a job to their best ability. I think it's taken on different meanings to what it probably had when it was first coined for somebody who was in a professional [*six seconds*] position.

Int. 26 offers a similar line of reasoning to that of Int. 22. However, he also displayed tendencies towards using the term professionalism to evidence that he has done a good job or offered a good service. When asked to define the term professionalism, he found it somewhat vexing, and used professional and professionalism interchangeably:

> [*Eighteen seconds*] Professionalism I would say is erm [*seven seconds*] is about err, doing [*seven seconds*] doing a good job, doing a job erm [*25 seconds*] yeah, to the best; it's hard isn't it, to define actually? But you talk about doing things in a professional way [*eight seconds*] erm [*nine seconds*] it's about err [*nine seconds*] [*blows air*] [*eight seconds*] being calm, being you know, presenting erm a good, always presenting a good face to students, and colleagues, erm it's about erm keeping up-to-date I think erm [*30 seconds*]. I'm struggling with that.

However, Int. 16 gave the most interesting, amusing, and questionable definition of a professional (despite him being the eldest respondent with over 30 years of service) when he said:

> Oh God! No! [*waving his hands about in a frantic manner*]. The answer to that question is no [*starts laughing*]. Erm [*five seconds*] ... it's like a duck, you'll know it if you see it.

Nevertheless, despite teaching human resource management, and being a member of the Chartered Institute of Personnel and Development (CIPD), Int. 16 could not offer a clear definition of the term. In fact, all of the 26 interviewees had problems defining a professional, often opting to define professionalism, including those who had just undertaken an assignment on the subject as part of their Postgraduate Certificate in Education (PGCE) qualification assessment. For example, Int. 5 stated:

> [*Laughs*] I've just written an assignment on it ... [*still laughing*] I should know, erm [*seven seconds*] to me [*four seconds*] being a professional ... erm [*six seconds*] is [*eight seconds*]; don't know, it's hard not to think of all the definitions that I've gone through in the past [*six seconds*] three weeks. Erm [*four seconds*] but to me it's somebody who's [*seven seconds*] qualified to do the job [*eight seconds*] erm [*six seconds*] ... who erm [*seven seconds*] is allowed, is somebody who has the, the freedom to do the job [*four seconds*] without constant, you know? You, you have the autonomy to do [*six seconds*] the job that you think, you know, you're trusted to do the job. Erm without referring it on [*four seconds*] erm [*five seconds*], but in, in return for that you do things, like you keep yourself up to date, erm [*five seconds*] you [*11 seconds*] ... I don't know, I suppose it's, it's a two-way street. You get the autonomy, but in return, you have to do the job. Erm [*six seconds*] and if, if you don't, I wouldn't, although

you might [referring to me as a lecturer employed by a HE institution] [*five seconds*] by street definition be classed as a professional, I wouldn't see that person if he just comes and doesn't do it [the job] as a professional.

From these observations from the lecturers interviewed, common themes manifested were those of relationships with students and colleagues, autonomy, service, trust, keeping up-to-date with materials, doing a good job, and being qualified.

On qualifications, Clow (2001) argues that due to the diversity of FE lecturer qualifications and experience, FE qualifications may be found somewhat wanting, in comparison to those of law and medicine. As such, this may suggest that FE lecturers may be viewed as not having, or belonging to, a profession. However, this changed in April 2008 when the Institute for Learning (IFL) became the official recognised professional body for lecturers teaching in FECs (Feather 2009). This professional body has similar powers as those for law and medicine, and therefore, any lecturer not complying with the ruling that they undertake 30 hours of continuous professional development (CPD) per year (Clancy 2007) may not be allowed to teach until they have amassed the necessary 30 hours and recorded it with the IFL (Heath 2007; IFL 2008; Feather 2009; Gale, Turner, and McKenzie 2011). This trend is further warranted when, as Clancy (2007, 2) writes, 'Like teachers in schools, lecturers in colleges are now required to register with the professional body and face being struck off for failing to uphold a code of behaviours'.

Professionalism: a Janus identity

Bathmaker and Avis (2005b, 5) argue that professionalism has two tiers:

> Within the literature, those who seek opportunities for transformative democratic practices and critical pedagogies distinguish between forms of professional identity which involve compliance with performative requirements of management cultures, and professional identities which are defined as 'authentic' to democratic values and practices.

One could argue from this perspective that professionalism is a 'Janus' identity in that one face depicts a professional who is said to be a person that complies with the practices laid down by management (Feather 2009), as depicted by the term managerialism (see Churchman 2002; Wynyard 2002; Ball 2003; Beck and Young 2005; Hodkinson 2008; Deem, Hillyard, and Reed 2010). The second face is one that holds true to the authentic practices built up over time (Feather 2009) and does not focus on targets, but instead focuses on democracy, and ensuring that people's values are taken into consideration; something akin to what Int. 8 said above about integrity and honesty. Harris (2005, 425) may be in accord with this when writing 'professionals are caught between, what they refer to as, the "economy of performance" and the "ecologies of practice".' Int. 11 relates to this when he is defining a professional, saying:

> From my point of view, it's erm, having a set of core values, erm, a set of ethics, erm, self-regulating, and time to, erm, reflect, time to research, erm [*six seconds*] in some ways erm [*four seconds*] putting the client before yourself. But it's also, it also means erm, respect from others, respect from the management, and erm, adequate remuneration...There's being an awful lot, well since incorporation, erm, was it 1993, or sometime like that, where, where erm, colleges were [*10 seconds*] became run more like a business. I mean this is, this is, this is serious business [*five seconds*] erm, I mean it's

run by business people in this college. Erm, the, the learners, or the [*four seconds*] or what we call, we call the learners, but it's actually the funding that the learners bring that is central to what we do. So erm, professionalism has to take a back seat, to, to erm, what is in effect a moneymaking business now. But it's [*seven seconds*] I mean, we find ourselves [*nine seconds*] we find ourselves erm, pressured to get your three Rs – recruitment, retention and results – and that final 10 percent of whatever funding. Erm, you know, there's a lot of pressure, a lot of pressure to err, to do that.

This then reflects Shain's (1998) views of teaching being deprofessionalised by management and management philosophies. In this respect, the teacher's professional status is to be laid to one side in order to focus on other issues. Int. 9 echoed the above, and became quite angry about how various stakeholders were now influencing professionalism within his particular FEC:

Everything's government, to do with the funding and support. Now there's no room to manoeuvre in any way, so, got to have simply one direction, and no moving sideways. So therefore, I think people can't run out, from our, from the professions itself, because they cannot cope with the expectations from the government, from the funders, from the people of the community, and so on. So in a way it's loosely fixed on meaning … in a way, and not only that, I think [*three seconds*] if you look at the position of the teachers themselves, might, if we take a [*six seconds*] the students as customers for example, they have more power now, and if for the teachers their hands are tied … So the profession says lose its meaning, because it doesn't have the power, they're all tied. So in other words, you do things as you've been told, because they're created [*five seconds*] the more students you've got the more money you're gonna have. So even in terms of, you're looking for numbers, not looking for quality of the students, it's the quantity, so in other words, people are moving towards business rather than to do teaching itself.

These views then appear to resonate with the ideas put forward by Bathmaker and Avis (2005b), and Harris (2005) earlier. This then offers some viability to the idea that professionalism is Janus-faced. Perhaps the most serious disadvantage of this suggestion is that individuals cannot physically split into two people. Therefore, they may choose to go with the compliance route, or with retaining the traditional values laid down by the profession. However, there may be a darker side to this that one must take into consideration. That is, people can have a number of 'selfs' (Solomon 1994; Barnett 2003), and as such may learn, and give off signals that they belong to one camp, whilst in reality they belong to another, or both. Hofstede and Hofstede (2005) call this 'political acting' and/or 'mental programming'. These multiple selfs, will in part, be exhibited when immersed in a particular habitus (Bourdieu 1988), or imaginary space (Clegg 2008). Having said this, a further problem presents itself in that a person could suffer with role conflict (Colbeck 1998), or, like Schön (2002) suggests, a person in the teaching profession might find their self in conflict with their individual values and beliefs, or if their values and beliefs are out of kilter with those of the habitus they are occupying, or working in. Int. 25 observed that she did change her professional stance depending on where she was teaching at any given time: 'Making sure that you're complying with the organisation's own standards … so there would be a certain format. I mean I find that, depending on who I'm teaching for … what they expect to see, varies enormously.' Int. 17, also identified that his personal values and beliefs were out of kilter with those of the organisation, and as such, he made 'choices' about what he was going to do:

I think the problem is that the government always wants everything done a little bit cheaper, and that actually [*drags word out*] [*eight seconds*] so we come back to that awful problem of [*four seconds*] as soon as we limit things by cost, we actually probably compromise what is achievable. I do think [*six seconds*] a lot of what goes on is done on the basis of good will. I know many colleagues who regularly (happily), work up to 60 hours a week; that is not for me. Erm, personal reasons, long period off, heart problem; so I'm not going to repeat that exercise at all. I'm limiting what I do, but that actually ... perhaps will that make me less professional?

From the above it has become evident that the terms professional and professionalism are indeed complex, and the qualitative data presented here has identified that the term professional is now a common, possibly overused, everyday term; to such an extent that it may have lost some of its original meaning. It appears that the term is Janus-faced – where one face sees the individual sticking to the traditional views of the profession, and another sees individuals complying with the management or organisation's policies and procedures. To this end, because of pressures placed upon them by their management, some individuals like Int. 17 are looking to his own values and beliefs, and to his health. As he identified, this may compromise the service he delivers. The inference here is that if these pressures are affecting him and others I interviewed, it may be the same for lecturers in other institutions. One example of this comes from my earlier (Feather 2009) work, where I identified that some lecturers were delivering HE at the FE level.

Conclusion

The paper has shown that to try to define the terms professional and professionalism is almost an insurmountable task, mainly due to their complexity and subjectivity. The perspectives of various authors have been discussed in this paper and a brief overview of professionalism has been provided.

A number of themes emerged from the study – those of behaviour; respect; autonomy; relationships with students and colleagues; codes of practice; doing a good job; service; qualifications; and keeping up-to-date with materials. From this, many of the lecturers interviewed held to their own perceived code of expected behaviour, in what they perceived to be professional, or adapted their professional behaviour (for better or worse) to fit in with the community they were working in.

Since 2008, lecturers in FECs in the UK have had to comply with the UK government's request to be members of the IFL (Clancy 2007), a professional body which has powers akin to those professional bodies of law and medicine. This means that if a lecturer does not comply with the standards laid down by the IFL they can be struck off from teaching in FECs until they have addressed the issues, for example, not attaining the 30 hours of CPD each year that lecturers are expected to undertake, record, and submit to the IFL (IFL 2008; Feather 2009).

When discussing professional standards it was identified that there may be two elements to professionalism (Bathmaker and Avis 2005b; Harris 2005), and therefore professionalism could be viewed as Janus-faced. One of these faces is seen as that of complying with new managerialist philosophies. Whereas the other face, the true face of professional/professionalism, adheres to the democratic core values and beliefs of that profession, which has been built up and developed over time by the lecturers themselves. It was shown that some of those interviewed were actually endeavouring to comply with both, that is, they were displaying role conflict, and as such could be said to be, in some part, 'political actors' (Hofstede and Hofstede 2005), where they give off the signals of both elements, but are not true members of either.

Finally, many of those interviewed felt that their individual professionalism was being eroded by the demands placed upon their individual institutions by the government, and in turn on them by their managers; this is in line with the views of Shain (1998), Churchman (2002), and Churchman and King (2009). From this, some lecturers interviewed were quite open about how they were compromising on the quality of their teaching in order to meet the targets and audit culture they felt they were now immersed in, and in some institutions were delivering HE at the FE level. It was their belief that their individual FECs were more focused on obtaining funding and the quantity of students, than on the core element of their business – that of teaching, specialism and knowledge. To this end, their belief was that their individual institutions were acting more like businesses than institutions of learning.

The management of FECs needs to take a step back from the highly competitive arena that education has been thrust into by successive UK governments, and examine their practices to ensure that their staff and students' needs are being taken into account when implementing new policies from government. Management need to remember that their frontline staff (lecturers) are the customer-facing staff, and need to be highly motivated both intrinsically and extrinsically. Not all motivation is about money; it can be, as many of the lecturers interviewed stated, 'the little things in life'. For example a thank you, or time to study and improve their knowledge – one of the key elements of professionalism identified by Perkin (2002), Mintzberg (1993), and Archer (2008). Those lecturers I spoke with were very passionate about their professionalism and the work they do; to them being a professional or acting professionally was about 'doing a good job!' They are professionals; management need to acknowledge this.

References

Archer, Margaret. S. 2000. *Being Human – the Problem of Agency.* Cambridge: Cambridge University Press.

Archer, Louise. 2008. "Younger Academics' Construction of 'Authenticity', 'Success' and Professional Identity." *Studies in Higher Education* 33 (4): 383–403. doi:10.1080/03075070802211729.

Ball, Stephen. J. 2003. "The Teacher's Soul and the Terrors of Performativity." *Journal of Education Policy* 18 (2): 215–228. doi:10.1080/0268093022000043065.

Barnett, Ronald. 2003. *Beyond All Reason – Living with Ideology in the University.* Buckingham: SRHE and Open University Press.

Bathmaker, Ann-Marie, and James Avis. 2005a. "Becoming a Lecturer in Further Education in England: The Construction of Professional Identity and the Role of Communities of Practice." *Journal of Education for Teaching* 31 (1): 47–62. doi:10.1080/02607470500043771.

Bathmaker, Ann-Marie, and James Avis. 2005b. "Is That 'Tingling Feeling' Enough? Constructions of Teaching and Learning in Further Education." *Educational Review* 57 (1): 3–20. doi:10.1080/0013191042000274150.

Bayer, A. E., and J. M. Braxton. 1998. "The Normative Structure of Community College Teaching: A Marker of Professionalism." *The Journal of Higher Education* 69 (2): 187–205. doi:10.2307/2649205.

Beck, John, and Michael F. D. Young. 2005. "The Assault on the Professions and the Restructuring of Academic and Professional Identities: A Bernsteinian Analysis." *British Journal of Sociology of Education* 26 (2): 183–197. doi:10.1080/0142569042000294165.

BERA. 2003. "BERA – Good Practice in Educational Research Writing." British Education Research Association. Accessed January 13, 2008. www.bera.ac.uk/publications/pdfs/GOODPR1.PDF

BERA. 2011. "Ethical Guidelines for Educational Research." BERA. Accessed September 29, 2013. http://www.bera.ac.uk/publications/guides.php

Bourdieu, Pierre. 1988. *Homo Academicvs*. Translated by P. Collier. Cambridge: Polity Press.

Castells, Manuel. 2010. *The Power of Identity – the Information Age: Economy, Society, and Culture*, Vol. II. Chichester: John Wiley and Sons.

Churchman, Deborah. 2002. "Voices of the Academy: Academics' Responses to the Corporatizing of Academia." *Critical Perspectives on Accounting* 13 (5–6): 643–656. doi:10.1006/cpac. 2002.0564.

Churchman, Deborah, and Sharon King. 2009. "Academic Practice in Transition: Hidden Stories of Academic Identities." *Teaching in Higher Education* 14 (5): 507–516. doi:10.1080/13562510903186675.

Clancy, Joe. 2007. "Checklist for the Model Profession." *The Guardian*, October 9.

Clegg, Sue. 2008. "Academic Identities under Threat?" *British Educational Research Journal* 34 (3): 329–345. doi:10.1080/01411920701532269.

Clow, R. 2001. "Further Education Teachers' Constructions of Professionalism." *Journal of Vocational Education and Training* 53 (3): 407–419. doi:10.1080/13636820100200166.

Colbeck, C. L. 1998. "Merging in a Seamless Blend: How Faculty Integrated Teaching and Research." *Journal of Higher Education* 69 (6): 647–671. doi:10.2307/2649212.

Deem, Rosemary, Sam Hillyard, and Mike Reed. 2010. *Knowledge, Higher Education, and the New Managerialism – the Changing Management of UK Universities*. Oxford: Oxford University Press.

Denscombe, Martyn. 2012. *The Good Research Guide for Small-scale Social Research Projects*. 4th ed. Maidenhead: Open University Press.

Farrugia, Charles. 1996. "A Continuing Professional Development Model for Quality Assurance in Higher Education." *Quality Assurance in Education* 4 (2): 28–34. doi:10.1108/09684889610116030.

Feather, Denis. 2009. "Academic Identities: Voices from the Edge." Doctoral thesis, The Business School, University of Huddersfield, Huddersfield.

Feather, Denis. 2011a. "Culture of HE in FE – Exclave or Enclave?" *Research in Post-Compulsory Education* 16 (1): 15–30.

Feather, Denis. 2011b. "Oh to be a Scholar – an HE in FE Perspective." *Journal of Further and Higher Education* 36 (2): 243–261.

Friedson, Eliot. 2001. *Professionalism – the Third Logic*. Cambridge: Polity Press.

Gale, K., R. Turner, and L. M. McKenzie. 2011. Communites of Praxis? Scholarship and Practice Styles of the HE in FE Professional. *Journal of Vocational Education and Training* 63 (2): 159–169. doi:10.1080/13636820.2011.572175.

Gleeson, Denis, Jennifer Davies, and Eunice Wheeler. 2005. "On the Making and Taking of Professionalism in the Further Education Workplace." *British Journal of Sociology of Education* 26 (4): 445–460. doi:10.1080/01425690500199818.

Goodhall, Amanda. H. 2009. *Socrates in the Boardroom*. Woodstock: Princeton University Press.

Hall, Donald E. 2002. *The Academic Self – an Owner's Manual*. Columbus: The Ohio State University Press.

Harris, Suzy. 2005. "Rethinking Academic Identities in Neo-Liberal Times." *Teaching in Higher Education* 10 (4): 421–433. doi:10.1080/13562510500238986.

Heath, Lindsay. 2007. "Developing a Code of Conduct and Disciplinary Processes for the Institute for Learning." *InTuition* (Spring): 1–24.

Hodkinson, Phil. 2008. "Scientific Research, Educational Policy, and Educational Practice in the United Kingdom: The Impact of the Audit Culture on Further Education." *Cultural Studies* 8 (3): 302–324.

Hofstede, Geert, and Gert Jan Hofstede. 2005. *Cultures and Organizations – Software of the Mind*. 2nd ed. London: McGraw-Hill.

IfL. 2008. "Member Handbook Version 2." Institute for Learning. Accessed July 26, 2008. www.ifl.ac.uk

Meek, V. Lynn. 1988. "Organizational Culture: Origins and Weaknesses." *Organisation Studies* 9 (4): 453–473. doi:10.1177/017084068800900401.

Mintzberg, Henry. 1993. *Structure in Fives – Designing Effective Organizations*. London: Prentice Hall International.

Nagy, Judy, and Tony Burch. 2009. "Communities of Practice in Academe (CoP-IA): Understanding Academic Work Practices to Enable Knowledge Building Capacities in Corporate Universities." *Oxford Review of Education* 35 (2): 227–247. doi:10.1080/03054980902792888.

Nixon, Jon. 2001. "'Not without Dust and Heat': The Moral Bases of the 'New' Academic Professionalism." *British Journal of Educational Studies* 49 (2): 173–186. doi:10.1111/1467-8527.00170.

Nixon, J., A. Marks, S. Rowland, and M. Walker. 2001. "Towards a New Academic Professionalism: A Manifesto of Hope." *British Journal of Sociology of Education* 22 (2): 227–244. doi:10.1080/01425690124202.

Parry, Gareth, and Anne Thompson. 2002. "Closer by Degrees – the Past, Present and Future of Higher Education in Further Education Colleges." Learning and Skills Development Agency, R1164/04/02/2200. LSDA. Accessed October 14, 2006. www.LSDA.org.uk

Perkin, Harold. 2002. *The Rise of Professional Society: England since 1880*. London: Routledge.

Robson, Colin. 2002. *Real World Research*. 2nd ed. Oxford: Blackwell.

Saunders, Mark, Philip Lewis, and Adrian Thornhill. 2007. *Research Methods for Business Students*. 4th ed. Harlow: Pearson Education.

Schön, Donald A. 2002. *The Reflective Practitioner – How Professionals Think in Action*. Ashford: Ashgate.

Schuck, Sandy, Sue Gordon, and John Buchanan. 2008. "What Are We Missing Here? Problematising Wisdoms on Teaching Quality and Professionalism in Higher Education." *Teaching in Higher Education* 13 (5): 537–547. doi:10.1080/13562510802334772.

Shain, Farzana. 1998. "Changing Notions of Teacher Professionalism in the Further Education Sector." Paper read at the British Educational Research Association Annual Conference, Queen's University of Belfast, Belfast, Northern Ireland, June 29.

Silver, H. 2003. "Does a University Have a Culture?" *Studies in Higher Education* 28 (2): 157–169. doi:10.1080/0307507032000058118.

Simmons, Jonathan. 2003. "Developing an 'HE Culture' in FE." Paper read at the 7th Annual LSRN Conference, Round Table Discussion, Coventry, December 10.

Solomon, Michael R. 1994. *Consumer Behaviour*. London: Allyn and Bacon.

Teddlie, Charles, and Abbaa Tashakkori. 2009. *Foundations of Mixed Methods Research*. London: Sage.

Turner, Rebecca, Liz McKenzie, and Mark Stone. 2009. "'Square Peg – Round Hole': The Emerging Professional Identities of HE in FE Lecturers Working in a Partner College Network in South-West England." *Research in Post-Compulsory Education* 14 (4): 355–368. doi:10.1080/13596740903360919.

Wolf, Alison. 2011. "Review of Vocational Education – the Wolf Report." Department for Education, DFE-00031-2011. HMSO. Accessed August 21, 2011. www.education.gov.uk/publications/.../The%20Wolf%20Report.pdf

Wynyard, Robin. 2002. "Hamburgerology by Degrees." In *The McDonaldization of Higher Education*, edited by D. Hayes and R. Wynyard, 200–210. London: Bergin and Garvey.

Locating post-16 professionalism: public spaces as dissenting spaces

Carol Azumah Dennis

Locating post-16 professionalism explores the ways in which teachers in the UK and the USA engaged in digitally mediated communication incidentally narrate their professional selves during extended exchanges about the process of post-qualification registration. Drawing on a theoretical framework derived from participatory democracy, the study is mindful of how citizens in public spaces express support or opposition to government policies. During their extended and intense discussion, the teachers involved discuss who legitimately defines and what justifiably bestows professional status. The paper is intent on questioning the location of professionalism rather than its definition. This spatial dimension is central to the argument that unfolds. Teacher professionalism is most frequently positioned within the classroom; a space that was once conceived as offering scope for strategic compliance. More recently, the classroom has become conceptualised as a diminutive space enabling of little more than teacher survival through tactical resistance. My argument is that teacher professionalism may also be located in other spaces, spaces that allow teachers to transcend the scripted pedagogies of the classroom. In these other spaces, teacher professionalism is located within open critique, defiance and dissent, which allow teachers to extend their pedagogic focus and explore dimensions of professionalism that matter to them: what it means, how and by whom it is conferred.

The classroom: an introduction

This paper argues that teacher professionalism may be located within spaces that allow teachers to transcend the diminutive space of the classroom in which teacher agency is proscribed. Through open critique, defiance and dissent, the contributors to these spaces extend the pedagogic focus to explore what it means to be a professional, how professionalism is conferred, and what it means to be considered as a professional. Such spaces extend and surround the pedagogic encounter. That is, the lives, experiences and histories of what it is like to be a teacher are suggested as locations that allow explicit critical articulation of what matters for teacher professionalism and provide a basis for where and how their professionalism may be located. The data that generated this discussion are located within the public domain – spaces that allow teachers (or more precisely, those who present themselves as teachers) to transcend the limitations of geographical location while simultaneously establishing extended and engaged contact with interested audiences who share their concerns. The analysis draws on the theoretical framework of participatory democracy. This reading emphasises the extent to which citizens who are involved and interested in teaching collaboratively and actively participate in the shaping of a response to an aspect of public policy – the process through which someone becomes qualified and recognised as a professional teacher. A participatory democracy framework is particularly fitting for data located within an inherently public domain (an online staffroom associated with a national newspaper) and an open discussion thread following a newspaper report about a group of protesting teachers. Those who contribute towards these spaces are participating in a public and political domain. Participatory democracy is mindful of how citizens express support or opposition to public policies. The specific focus in this paper is educational policy, with a particular interest in the process of professional recognition.

It is not my intention to further define teacher professionalism. These uncertainties are well-rehearsed and can be revisited elsewhere (Bathmaker and Avis 2005; Dennis 2010; Robson 1998; Stronach et al. 2002). Instead, I explore how those with an interest in teaching or who present themselves as teachers engage in digitally mediated communication incidentally, articulating a notion of professionalism in the process of online exchange about an important aspect of public policy. In referring to 'teacher' I am keen to avoid my analysis becoming embroiled within a peripheral evaluation of possible nomenclatures associated with those who work within different educational settings: trainer, facilitator, lecturer, learning support. 'Teacher' establishes a shared discourse that accommodates the privileged analytical status I offer to those who work in further education, while nonetheless drawing on literatures derived from schools, adult and higher education.

My argument is that spaces of public dissent are spaces within which it is possible to locate teacher professionalism (Dewey 2012; Stitzlein and Quinn 2012, 191). In these spaces, contributors publicise their professional knowledge and expose overlooked problems in public policy. Contributors also express their views, highlighting in and for the public important matters of concern. This is more than angry emotional outpourings. It is a forum for the activist professional (Groundwater-Smith and Sachs 2002) to rally support for a cause. Contributors to such spaces re-envision professionalism, offering not only improved or alternative processes, but, more broadly, an alternative construct for the place and purpose of teacher professionalism.

The paper positions itself within a global research imagination (Kenway and Fahey 2009, 1). In so doing, I place alongside each other two disparate interactions, involving post-16 teachers in the UK as they engage in dissenting discussion about professional body membership and professional formation, and graduating teachers from a university in the USA as they discuss the process through which they achieve post-qualification professional recognition. This placing alongside each other is premised upon recognising that both sets of dissenting teachers are caught up within a maelstrom of what some refer to as the neoliberal assault on education. What emerge are critical engagements through which teachers engage – at times reflexively – with how professionalism is understood – by themselves and by policy – and the basis upon which it is conferred.

Mapping spaces of dissent

Surrounding teachers in post-16 education are a series of axial tensions between professional aspiration and policy embodiment (Dennis 2012). Teachers' professional identities emerge from how they negotiate policy requirements and professional commitments. This is a space within which practitioners comply with policy, but their compliance is outward, superficial and strategic (Shain and Gleeson 1999).

Orr (2011) has revisited this idea of strategic compliance and suggested that it is an outdated analysis of what it is like to work within a contemporary post-16 college. Ongoing managerial incursions into what was once regarded as the autonomous locus of control for the professional have been so relentlessly extreme that space for manoeuvrability has been eroded. Teachers are just about able to cope within an environment that is increasingly threatening not only to their professionalism, but also to their wellbeing. Within these constraints, teachers do little more than survive; rather than being strategic, their negotiating space is at best defined as tactical. Skirmishes with managerialism are short-term and opportunistic, with no ultimate goal beyond the immediate. Orr's analysis is troubling and his re-mapping resonates. The professional locus of control, once strategic in scope, is now constricted within the diminutive space of the sealed classroom. This conceptualisation betrays an impoverished conception of professional pedagogic spaces. It negates teachers' and those that surround them, the capacity for situated, embodied, critical reflexivity and praxis. If teaching is indeed a profession, the task is to locate that professionalism, not as something which is here or there, but rather as something that folds into the pedagogic space of the classroom. This folding into is explored here. My argument is that these are spaces within which teachers care for their professional selves. They 'think in terms of what they [do and] do not want to be, and [do and] do not want to *become*' (Ball and Olmedo 2013, 86, original emphasis). These spaces fold back into and become part of the pedagogic encounter. They are what teachers bring with them to that encounter.

Methodology: what do teachers talk about when they talk amongst themselves?

The first space explored is the *Times Educational Supplement* (TES) (TES Community 2013). The *Times Educational Supplement*, a UK-based national newspaper, hosts an online teachers' staffroom. It is a password-protected forum, open to all who have access to email and choose to register after agreeing to legally binding terms and conditions. There is no scope to verify the identity of those who contribute postings, and so when I refer to 'teachers' I might more meaningfully refer to 'those who present themselves as teachers'. The TES online staffroom is described by themselves as the: 'World's biggest teaching community. Where teachers can get together with teachers from around the world who can offer classroom support, healthy debate and a whole lot of inspiration' (TES Community 2013). This space was selected because it is unique in the UK. There is no comparative public online space in the UK that brings together such a disparate group of loosely affiliated professionals for publicly available extended policy and practice discussion. The absolute identity of contributors remains ambiguous as they might be other than they suggest. However, the material explored here is the discursive content and context of their discussion rather than the identity and motivation of those who contribute.

The second source of data is an online readers' response forum associated with a newspaper in the USA, *The New York Times* (Winerip 2012). There is no password protection required to enter this moderated space.

New posts and new threads for discussion are opened or closed on the TES site on a daily basis. At the time of this enquiry, there were 114 different threads on varying subjects. Counting only those threads with more than 10 comments, there were 2800 different contributions. My analysis focuses on a thread entitled, 'Should we keep the professional body in business?' This space was selected for closer analysis because it was clearly the most frequently visited of the 114 forums. 'Should we keep the professional body in business?' focuses around whether post-16 teachers in the UK should comply with the legislative requirement to pay membership fees to a state-sponsored professional body. My analysis starts with the opening of the thread in May 2010 and ends with its closing in December 2012. Those who contribute to these discussions have defined what is important and interesting and in need of discussion for themselves. They are not responding to a researcher-initiated concern. 'Should we keep the professional body in business?' attracted 225 contributions, in contrast to other discussion threads, which attracted in the region of 60 contributions. The 225 different comments were posted by 60 different contributors, 32 of whom made 2 or more comments over the 2 years. The most prolific commentator had 30 different postings. There were 28 commentators who made only 1 contribution. Each comment averaged at 110 words. 'Should we keep the professional body in business?' was clearly a highly engaging matter of concern.

The user-generated content in response to a newspaper story in the USA was selected after a careful review of online forums in newspapers devoted to education and teachers or with stories of interest to and relevance for professionalisation. 'Move to outsource' was selected on the basis that it focused on the same subject as 'Should we keep the professional body in business?' and had a substantial number of detailed comments associated with it. There were 79, rather than 60, different contributors to the discussion. My analysis follows the opening and closing of user-generated responses. The newspaper story appeared on 6 May 2012 (Winerip 2012). Within two days, the article had generated 79 comments at which point the comments section was closed by the newspaper. Each posting averaged 100 words. Few posters commented more than once and most contributions refer directly to the featured story.

In 'Move to outsource' (Winerip 2012), the featured comments offer links to other online spaces, where discussion continues. The teachers who form the basis of the news story elaborate upon and articulate their motivation as part of two, hour-long group interviews on a community radio station devoted to critical education (Madeloni, Keisch Polin, and Scott 2012). A digital recording of these interviews is hosted on a blog that features more detailed discussion and commentary about the newspaper story and the ongoing concerns it generates.

While online spaces have strong capacity to nurture dissent, they are also able to mimic the exclusions and silences that appear in other aspects of professional life (DiMaggio et al. 2004). In arguing these spaces as the location for openly critical, defiant and dissenting teacher professionalism, I treat them as a source of illustrative data rather than an analytical object in possession of inherent qualities.

These data raise ethical dilemmas. The distinction between public and private (Driscoll and Gregg 2010) blurs uncomfortably, giving rise to important questions about informed consent and confidentiality. I treat this written talk-in-interaction as text. The method used does not directly involve contact with a human subject and the question of informed consent is inflected rather than irrelevant. There has been no direct exchange between myself as researcher and any of the online posters. At least six months elapsed between the final contribution and the start of my analysis. I have explored digital footprints available in a public domain (Thorseth 2003), albeit one that requires access to email. The stance I have taken is consistent with that proposed by the British Educational Research Association and the Association of Internet Researchers (AoIR) (Markham and Buchanan 2012). The AoIR advise that the more an online space is accepted as public, the less likely it is that research will intrude upon the privacy, confidentiality and right to informed consent of the individuals involved (Ess and the AoIR Ethics Working Group, cited by Jones 2011).

The public nature of these data is further emphasised by their hyperlinked intertextuality. The TES online staffroom, 'Should we keep the professional body in business?', consists of an extensive posting and a multiple authored and signatured letter published in a national newspaper. The space is explicitly used to gather support in the form of signatures to a campaigning letter. Extracts from the forum regularly appear in the TES. What I am careful to establish here is the expectation each contributor might reasonably have about the privacy, confidentiality and further use of their online musings, even if these musings are part of a gift economy. The data have been used with the permission of the TES, who ask contributors to relinquish copyright as part of their terms and conditions of use.

My suggestion is that post-16 teachers' professionalism may be located within an exploration of these online spaces; within spaces that are significant enfoldings of the pedagogic encounter. In these spaces, teachers are able to extend the possibilities of the diminutive classroom that enables only tactical resistance. They engage in open, exploratory, dissenting critique.

'Should we keep the professional body in business?' is a dissenting space; while specific contributions may or may not be supportive of the professional body, the thread itself assumes a dissenting stance. Membership of the professional body was not a matter of preference. It was a legal obligation. The thread's title, a question, implies choice and, as such, conveys the possibility at least of defiance. The discursive reference to 'business' positions teachers as customers who may or may not support a profit-making enterprise. 'Move to outsource' is an intensely focused analytical space that takes place over a shorter period of time. A newspaper article is followed by comments in which each contributor clearly indicates their support for those who boycott the professional registration process.

Method: coding, categorising and tabulating

The data are digital but this does not determine the mode of analysis, which resembled a six-phase recursive, iterative process. Successive re-readings gave me a feel for the tone, texture and shape of the data. This was followed up with my trying out of multiple approaches to coding and re-coding. Having identified particular points of interest, successive initial codings with numerous categories were subsumed into broader thematic codes as detailed below. Referring back to the overall purpose of the study then led to organising these within three main interrogations. This is what has guided how the data were finally written. A final search, review and clarification led to the selecting of major themes as they reappeared throughout the discussion and between the different sets of data.

My final analysis did not echo the thread's question 'Should we keep the professional body in business?' but, mindful that the question itself implies an answer (possibly not), instead focused on *why* – according to this forum – post-16 teachers *should not* keep the professional body in business or, in the case of 'Move to outsource', why recently qualified graduate teachers *should not* comply with the professional registration process. None of those who participate in the discussion reference participatory democracy. I have used participatory democracy as an overall conceptual framework to theorise the significance of these data. The data allow me to gain an insight into what teachers talk about when they talk amongst themselves. Compliance or non-compliance with professional formation is not the focus of my study. What I am exploring is how diminution of tactical resistance or a strategy of superficial compliance becomes open critique, defiance and dissent. The data feel like overheard staffroom conversations in which teachers say what they really think without reference to an externally defined agenda. My underlying intention is to consider what this implies for how teachers experience their professionalism.

I draw on data from the UK and the USA not to imply a smoothed-out sameness but, rather, to suggest a single point of similarity: teachers engaging with an unwelcome policy requirement for post-qualification professional recognition. This requirement emerges from a global educational policy nexus (Verger, Novelli, and Altinyelken 2012) that generates a particular view of education as located within a market rather than in a public sphere. Standardised processes commodify and, as such, standardisation creates the necessary conditions for creation of educational markets. A spatially aware, multi-layered approach to policy analysis, which places emphasis on relationality and interconnectivity (Rizvi and Lingard 2010), is central to understanding how educational desire is subsumed beneath the needs of the educational market.

Locating professionalism: what is wrong with a 'professional body'?

In July 2014, the professional body[1] for FE teachers in the UK announced it was set to close and transfer its assets to the Employment and Training Foundation, a Coalition government-instituted organisation that emerged following the Lingfield Review (Lingfield 2012) of standards in the sector. As a professional body for post-16 teachers in England, it was first instituted in 2002 and in the years that followed had a voluntary membership of about 2000 lecturers. In 2007, new regulations surrounding Further and Higher Education made membership of the professional body mandatory for all teachers working in post-16 provision. Individual membership fees, initially paid for by government on behalf of teachers, by 2012 were required from members to enable the professional body to become self-financing (Business, Innovation and Skills 2009). It is not the intention of this paper to assume a position in favour of or opposed to the continuation of a professional body for FE teachers. This was, and remains, hotly contested. The interest explored here is one of dissent in a public space analysed as significant within a theoretical framework of participatory democracy.

Throughout the TES forum 'Should we keep the professional body in business?' teachers felt they were being bullied into membership; indeed, in a survey conducted by the professional body, 47% had taken out professional membership against their wishes (Thomson 2008). An organisation that was instituted to protect their professional interests was requiring them to be 'milquetoasts, cowering in the corner' (TES Community 2013); that is, passive and weak in response to the impositions of policy.

'Should we keep the professional body in business?' revolves around an important and pronounced act of collective dissent by post-16 teachers in the UK.

In rejecting mandatory membership of a professional body, contributors were not rejecting the idea of themselves as professionals. A sense of professionalism was unanimously accepted as a powerful determinate of classroom conduct. Their rejection of the professional body was conditional. If professionalism is bestowed by virtue of joining a fee-paying organisation, then it should be a fee-paying organisation instigated by the members themselves, not one dictated by government:

> A true professional body would be created and controlled by the members. The professional body was created by the government on a whim, it is NOT representative of the members. (TES Forum, Crackers, TES Community 2013)[2]

The credibility of the professional body is questioned, as is the validity of conferring professional status through such membership. An underlying question is implied: who defines and what bestows professional status?

> The previous government quite rightly introduced legislation to make all post-16 teachers gain a recognised teaching qualification, such as a PGCE, CertEd or DTLLS ... which I possess, and surely this proves a lecturer as being 'qualified to teach'. I have myself been graded as 'outstanding', grade one, by both internal and external OfSTED inspections, who again regularly assess my abilities and competence. Yet even had I been graded as 'inadequate', grade four, I would still have been entitled to join the professional body, confirming my professionalism. (TES Forum, Crackers, TES Community 2013)

> I know I'm a trained professional and so do my colleagues. Perhaps they realise we are, in fact, recognised as professionals without needing this unnecessary additional tax on our chosen vocation? (TES Forum, Healthy Teacher, TES Community 2013)

The thread examines the practicalities of professional body membership – for a moment at least they sideline the principle at stake. They calculate in detail the cost implications for college budgets if fees were paid by employers. The implication is that they are prepared to tolerate belonging to a professional body if membership fees are paid on their behalf. The discussion of professional body membership is focused almost exclusively here around what contributors believe to be highly valued and appropriate conduct in the physicality of the classroom setting. Their analysis is premised upon defining who teachers are, and what they do – when teaching.

This is important because the discussion leads to other more fundamental reasons being cited for rejecting mandatory membership: its existence exposes an improper fit between post-16 teaching and the associated terms and conditions of service – the relationship between professional membership and professional status, the nature of policy imposition and what can legitimately be required from lecturers are all aspects of this debate. In weighing the cost and benefits of professional body membership, one contributor illustrates the divergent strands of thought:

> Those of us who have worked out that as part-timers we probably earn about £2 an hour after we have taken into account planning lessons and schemes of work, gathering information and resources, setting up PowerPoint presentations and other resources, monitoring and recording progress, writing reports, gathering data for our employers,

preparing to meet the strictures for the 'outstanding' lessons that class visitors wish to see, and – nearly forgot – actually teaching, are a tad emotional. (TES Forum, ZHC, TES Community 2013)

The teachers who rejected the professional body through this discussion thread coalesce around this view. It was not the idea of teaching as a profession that they were rejecting. What troubled was the idea that teachers who had undergone a period of academic qualification, who were respected by colleagues, who had demonstrated their commitment to developing valued classroom practices – sometimes to the detriment of their health and wellbeing, teachers who were in many instances poorly paid on insecure hour-by-hour contracts – were further imposed upon by the requirement that they pay a fee to a legislatively derived organisation to which they felt no allegiance. The classroom is central to their discussion.

Locating professionalism: who confers professional status?

Teachers of arts and crafts, languages, book clubs, family and local history, skills for life and so on, know that their efforts bring satisfaction, pleasure and wellbeing to hundreds of thousands of people. (TES Forum, DiOxide, TES Community 2013)

This contribution conveys an embodied, experiential, rather than an argumentative, truth. The contributor is arguing for a notion of teaching and learning that is not predicated upon the contribution it makes to the economic good. It is instead valued for the 'satisfaction, pleasure and well-being' it brings. New Labour's Skills for Life policy is an intriguing reference here. Between 2001 and 2010, Skills for Life exemplified New Labour's ideas about education as shifting from an adjunct to a direct focus for economic policy (Dennis 2010). Literacy and Numeracy provision were recast as strictly vocational, an economic good predicated upon global competition between states. Its grouping alongside curricular subjects associated with the liberal arts is both striking and casual. I suggest it marks a blasé refusal of policy-predicated determinations. That is, despite the entire weight of policy defining Literacy and Numeracy as skills required for global competition, the writer of this letter and her co-signatories blithely associate Skills for Life with the liberal arts, subjects that, if valued at all, are valued for entirely different reasons.

This is an emotive space. And contributors return to the thread's central theme: their professionalism is not secured through mandatory membership of a legislatively imposed body. Professional body membership was neither a necessary nor sufficient pre-requisite for professional status. Such membership could not compensate for other more pressing concerns, such as the terms and conditions of service:

[We are] the lowest of the low in the college hierarchy. 'The professional body' may try to tell you otherwise, but the reality is that teaching is much like serving burgers in a fast food outlet. That is: lowest cost to operate. (TES Forum, Healthy Teacher, TES Community 2013)

My intention here is not to interrogate the internal consistency or evidence base for the arguments put forward. It would also be misleading to suggest that the thread maintains a single line of argument. There are misconception, variation, incoherence and disagreement around professional body membership and all that it attends. My reading of this thread is based on following the divergent lines of argumentation that determine the oppositional stance taken. Amidst these exchanges, professionalism emerges as something that was self-derived, negotiated between professionals or a body of practitioners and the public. It was not something that was bestowed by policy. Nor for the experienced or qualified teacher was it located within policy-directed behaviour.

The focus of contributors' protests is a specific policy requirement, but at times their line of vision broadens. A casual resistance to the idea of education as handmaiden to the economy (Bates 1992) changes to connect the space of post-16 professionalism to discourses around equity, inclusion and social justice.

The space is an openly campaigning one. This is the text of a letter that later appeared in a national newspaper. It is posted in the forum in an attempt to gather more signatories:

> Opposition to the [mandatory membership of a professional body] fee is additionally symptomatic of a general malaise: the degradation of pay, conditions and pensions; the casualisation of part time and agency staff; issues of career development, pay differentials and promotion for women, Black, disabled and LGBT [lesbian, gay, bisexual and transexual] lecturers; the widening gulf between lecturers' pay and executive salaries; and the glaring inconsistencies in the wider sector's professionalism agenda with school teachers and HE lecturers. (TES Forum, Joel Petrie, TES Community 2013)

What emerges is a distinct sense of professionalism that is somehow preserved even when a teacher leaves their institutional moorings. In the following reference, a teacher without her actual teaching being observed, is graded as inadequate for not having the required paperwork with her on an unannounced observation. When informed she would be disciplined for gross professional misconduct, she decided to resign her post:

> I set up the classes privately, took the students along and almost immediately was taking home twice my previous hourly rate plus no hours of paperwork and no hassle from 'Management' (who were really just a bunch of über administrators suffering from OCD [obsessive-compulsive disorder]). As for the other post, I am whittling down the hours each year and hiring the halls privately. The students are happier and I feel more enthusiastic than I have in years. By September, I will only teach [a group of seriously disabled students to whom I feel very loyal]. (TES Forum, Entrepreneur, TES Community 2013)

There is no scope for verifying or refuting the account offered here. The reliability of the narrative and the appropriateness of either management's or the teacher's actions are not – in this analysis – significant. It is the independence of professional identity and the idea that even the physicality of the classroom can shift to accommodate the professional scope of the teacher that furthers my line of argument. Teacherly commitments to public service remain (in the form of commitment to the most vulnerable students) alongside a refusal to comply – strategically or tactically – with the administrative burden that she sees as imposing on her professionalism.

Locating professionalism: spaces for dissent

From 2007 to 2012, a regulated UK professional workforce required membership of a government-prescribed body and a time-bound target for newly appointed teachers to achieve Qualified Teacher in Learning and Skills (QTLS) status. Qualified Teacher in Learning and Skills status required the completion of a portfolio and reflective commentary, which, once assessed, formed the basis of full professional formation (IfL 2008). The suitability of the process itself did not significantly feature as part of the TES forum discussion. Discussion focused on the imposition of professional body membership. In the USA, the 'Move to outsource teacher licensing process' (Winerip 2012) features a university teacher educator and a group of recently qualified trainee teachers who refuse to participate in a pilot programme for a newly devised 'outsourced' licencing procedure developed by an international edu-business[3] (Ball 2012) in conjunction with Stanford University. The text does not reference which phase of education these graduates have qualified to teach. What connects 'Move to outsource' and 'Should we keep the professional body in business?' is that both protests articulate and defend professionalism as located within spaces other than those defined by policy. It is this insistence that allows the USA and the UK discussions to be analysed alongside each other as disparate instances of a closely connected phenomenon. The protests are heavily accented: a process, uncontested in the UK (the completion of a portfolio that is assessed at a distance and that allows professional status to be conferred), forms the basis of dispute in the USA. That similar policy processes of professional recognition have been deployed with post-16 teachers in the UK and with university graduate teachers in the USA is illustrative of the stretching of educational policy beyond the nation (Rizvi and Lingard 2010, 68). This study focuses on trans-local spaces, the detailed dissenting discussion between those who present themselves as teachers, as they attempt to resist the hegemonic power of the neoliberal imaginary. It is not my intention to overplay the commensurability of these spaces or the discussion that unfolds. A global awareness of educational policy need not imply smoothed-out sameness. The data derived from the US 'Move to outsource' illustrate an important dimension to my central line of argument, namely that teacher professionalism may be located within a public sphere. In such spaces, teachers draw on their knowledge to expose the problematics of policy; they rally for support and express solidarity; they also work alongside each other for political organisation. In these spaces, teachers participate in open critique, defiance and dissent. The analysis positions teachers as something other than the strategically compliant or tactically resistant self that occupies the diminutive space of the classroom. In these spaces, those who present themselves as teachers are also citizens who re-envision not only improved, but alternative, practices.

In 'Move to outsource' the main objection to a portfolio-based approach to conferring professional status (as required for QTLS in the UK) is that it implies a particular and unwelcome location for teacher professionalism. Compelled by competing gravitational centres, teacher professionalism may be located in the objective, standardised, codifiable space of the diminutive classroom. It is neatly bounded by acquired knowledge. It can be commodified, communicated and assessed at a distance. It can also be located within a market exchange – purchased – the licencing process in the USA required newly qualified teachers to pay in the region of $400. In the UK, the professional membership fee contributed towards the cost of professional formation. If teacher professionalism is located in this 'objective, standardised, codifiable' space, a portfolio can reasonably confer professional status and the licencing cost is justified.

Those who have refused participation in the outsourced licencing process argue that the assessment of teaching '… is something complex and we don't like seeing it taken out of human hands' (Winerip 2012). The forum is unanimous and contributors echo solidarity and support. Teacher professionalism is non-standardised, uncertain and situated. It is meaningful only when it is located within 'human hands'.

Once teaching and education are re-constructed along the lines articulated, paying a private company to confer professional status at a distance is argued as fundamentally flawed and unfit for purpose. Unable to confer professional status, the at-a-distance portfolio assessment enables the extraction of profit; profits accrued through public service contracts or direct fees charged to accrediting teachers. The process opens new territories of public life to private corporations.

Having constructed teacher professionalism as an inherently relational activity, the contributors to the forum question the derisory ways in which teachers are talked about in public discourse. This may seem to be a different and distinct conversational track to the licencing process, but it is closely connected. The at-a-distance process for conferring professional status bypassed teacher educators who in the policy imagination cannot be trusted to make a sound judgement. The contributors' analysis thus connects the physical activity of teaching to the licencing process, the denigration of teachers and teacher educators and an attempt to remove professionalism from the classroom into a competitive marketplace based on financial gain and exchange:

> The Holy Grail of 100% teacher competence and 100% student success is simply not achievable, and will not be realised by removing the responsibility and accountability of college professors, lead teachers, school boards, and school administrators to use their best judgement in selecting, supporting, and tenuring teaching candidates, and handing it over to a profit-driven monopoly, whose main allegiance is to its own bottom line. (*New York Times*, Delboy, Winerip 2012)

In refusing at-a-distance licencing, the protestors are refusing a delivery system that allows the bottom line to subsume educational values, needs and aspirations. They are asserting a belief in the value of education as a public good rather than an opportunity to secure private, profitable gain from public resources. The objective at-a-distance licencing process – with its primary focus on the bottom-line – bypasses democratic participation and accountability. It is what inevitably happens when an edu-business is answerable only to its shareholders. They:

> Do not answer to [those who represent students' interests]. And [those who represent students' interests] are given no choice about where the money goes. (*New York Times*, Brighton Spice, Winerip 2012)

The TES forum is less analytical about the implications of the professional body as corporate involvement in education. Though a single TES contributor does view the professional body as:

> ... a private company run for the benefit of its 'stakeholders' (which do not include compulsory members like us), and its main purpose seems ... money-making ... (TES Forum, Billy Rose, TES Community 2013)

Space for manoeuvrability: from strategic compliance to open dissent

In this paper, I have attempted to locate teacher professionalism rather than define it. I have acknowledged that while successive waves of educational reform have reduced teachers' scope for manoeuvrability from strategic compliance (Shain and Gleeson 1999) to tactical resistance (Orr 2011), discussion of teaching nonetheless continues in the public sphere in ways that allow those who identify themselves as teachers to articulate what they know about public policy and its limitations. They engage in extended analytical debate in order to rally support and solidarity, to raise awareness of their concerns and to cultivate the persona of an activist professional. In these spaces, those who represent themselves as teachers are openly critical, defiant and dissenting. They extend their pedagogic focus to explore what it means to be a professional, how their professionalism is conferred and the implications of their professionalism. I suggest that there are spaces of participatory democracy wherein those who represent themselves as teachers cultivate their values, beliefs and commitments. Professionalism might reasonably be located within these spaces.

What this implies is that there are professional spaces beyond those scripted by policy. In these public professional spaces, it is possible to locate a – practical, social and natural – world that is not wholly at the disposal of policy and might not obey its whims. There is an echo here of Meirieu's (2013) characterisation of policy approaches towards education as (at times) infantile: driven by the assumption that to declare the world is to define the world and thus to determine what can and what will happen in that world. The teachers in these spaces indicate otherwise. They can and do resist – and in so doing locate their professional selves. In these spaces, teacher professionalism is neither strategic nor tactical. It is instead argued as openly critical, defiant and dissenting. It is a professionalism that although located in public spaces of dissent, nonetheless folds back into the pedagogic encounter. What remains to be explored is in what other ways and what other spaces this openly critical, defiant and dissenting professionalism unfolds itself.

Disclosure statement

No potential conflict of interest was reported by the author.

Notes

1. The discussion revolves around the mandatory membership of the Institute for Learning in the UK. To maintain focus on professionalism (rather than the rights and wrongs of a particular organisation, the Institute for Learning) I have used the term 'professional body' throughout.
2. I have used pseudonyms rather than names as they appear in the thread. Although the material is available in the public domain, in re-contextualising it here, I have sought to offer some degree of anonymity.
3. I have avoided wherever possible explicit reference to the specific corporation involved as this is not central to the line of argument I am pursuing and may cause unnecessary distraction.

References

Ball, Stephen. 2012. *Global Education Inc: Policy Networks and Edu-Business*. London: Routledge.
Ball, Stephen, and A. Olmedo. 2013. "Care of the Self, Resistance and Subjectivity under Neoliberal Governmentalities." *Critical Studies in Education* 54 (1): 85–96.
Bates, R. 1992. "Educational Reform: Its Role in the Economic Destruction of Society." Keynote Address at the Joint Annual Meeting of the Australian Association of Research in Education and New Zealand Association of Research in Education, Geelong, VIC, Australia, November.

Bathmaker, A., and James Avis. 2005. "Becoming a Lecturer in Further Education in England: The Construction of Professional Identity and the Role of Communities of Practice." *Journal of Education for Teaching: International Research and Pedagogy* 31 (1): 47–62.

Business, Innovation and Skills. 2009. "Skills for Sustainable Growth | Policies | BIS." Accessed July 24, 2013. http://webarchive.nationalarchives.gov.uk/+/http://www.bis.gov.uk/skillsforgrowth

Dennis, Carol Azumah. 2010. "Is the Professionalisation of Adult Basic Skills Practice Possible, Desirable or Inevitable?" *Literacy and Numeracy Studies* 18 (2): 26–43.

Dennis, Carol Azumah. 2012. "Quality: An Ongoing Conversation over Time." *Journal of Vocational Education & Training* 64 (4): 511–527.

Dewey, J. 2012. *The Public and Its Problems: An Essay in Political Inquiry.* University Park, PA: Penn State University Press.

DiMaggio, P., E. Hargittai, C. Celeste, and S. Shafer. 2004. "Digital Inequality: From Unequal Access to Differentiated Use: A Literature Review and Agenda for Research on Digital Inequality." In *Social Inequality*, edited by Kathryn M. Neckerman, 355–400. New York: Russell Sage Foundation.

Driscoll, C., and M. Gregg. 2010. "My Profile: The Ethics of Virtual Ethnography." *Emotion, Space and Society* 3 (1): 15–20.

Groundwater-Smith, Susan, and Judyth Sachs. 2002. "The Activist Professional and the Reinstatement of Trust." *Cambridge Journal of Education* 32 (3): 341–358. http://dx.doi.org/10.1080/0305764022000024195

IfL (Institute for Learning). 2008. *Licence to Practise: Professional Formation. Your Guide to Qualified Teacher Learning and Skills (QTLS) and Associate Teacher Learning and Skills (ATLS) Status.* London: Author.

Jones, C. 2011. "Ethical Issues in Online Research." British Educational Research Association. Accessed July 23, 2013. http://www.bera.ac.uk/resources/ethical-issues-online-research

Kenway, J., and J. Fahey. 2009. "Imagining Research Otherwise." In *Globalizing the Research Imagination*, edited by J. Kenway and J. Fahey, 1–41. Abingdon: Routledge.

Lingfield, R. 2012. "Professionalism in Further Education. Interim Report of the Independent Review Panel." Accessed May 11, 2013. http://scholar.google.co.uk/scholar?hl=en&q=lingfield+professionalism&btnG=&as_sdt=1,5&as_sdtp=#0

Madeloni, B., D. Keisch Polin, and T. Scott. 2012. "Teacher Performance Assessment: A Money Grab for Pearson." *Education Radio: On Air.* Accessed November 23, 2013. http://education-radio.blogspot.co.uk/2012/03/teacher-performance-assessment-money.html

Markham, Annette, and Elizabeth Buchanan. 2012. *Ethical Decision-Making and Internet Research Recommendations from the AoIR Ethics Working Committee* (Version 2.0). Chicago, IL: Association of Internet Researchers. http://aoir.org/reports/ethics2.pdf

Meirieu, P. 2013. "Pédagogie: Le Devoir de Résister (2008) in Giving Teaching Back to Education: Responding to the Disappearance of the Teacher." *Phenomenology & Practice* 6 (2): 35–49.

Orr, K. 2011. "The End of 'Strategic Compliance'? Practice and Professionalism in the English Further Education Sector." Paper presented at the Journal of Vocational Education and Training Conference, Worcester College, Oxford, July 8–10. Unpublished.

Rizvi, F., and Bob Lingard. 2010. *Globalizing Education Policy.* London: Routledge.

Robson, J. 1998. "A Profession in Crisis: Status, Culture and Identity in the Further Education College." *Journal of Vocational Education and Training* 50 (4): 585–607.

Shain, F., and D. Gleeson. 1999. "Under New Management: Changing Conceptions of Teacher Professionalism and Policy in the Further Education Sector." *Journal of Education Policy* 14 (4): 445–462.

Stitzlein, Sarah M., and Sarah Quinn. 2012. "What Can We Learn from Teacher Dissent Online?" *The Educational Forum* 76 (2): 190–200. http://dx.doi.org/10.1080/00131725.2011.653870

Stronach, I., B. Corbin, O. McNamara, S. Stark, and T. Warne. 2002. "Towards an Uncertain Politics of Professionalism: Teacher and Nurse Identities in Flux." *Journal of Education Policy* 17 (1): 109–138.

TES Community. 2013. "Blogs, Forums and Groups for the World's Largest Education Community – TES Community." *Times Educational Supplement*. Accessed July 21, 2013. http://community.tes.co.uk/

Thomson, Alan. 2008. "Bullied into IfL Membership?" *Times Educational Supplement, FE News*. Accessed July 18, 2013. http://www.tes.co.uk/article.aspx?storycode=6005757

Thorseth, M. 2003. "Introduction." In *Applied Ethics in Internet Research*, edited by M. Thorseth, vii–xii. Trondheim, Norway: Norwegian University of Science and Technology.

Verger, Antoni, Mario Novelli, and Hülyu Kosa Altinyelken. 2012. "Global Education Policy and International Development: An Introductory Framework." In *Global Education Policy and International Development*, edited by Antoni Verger, Mario Novelli, and Hülyu Kosa Altinyelken, 3–31. London: Bloomsbury.

Winerip, Michael. 2012. "Move to Outsource Teacher Licensing Process Draws Protest." *New York Times*, May 6. http://www.nytimes.com/2012/05/07/education/new-procedure-for-teaching-license-draws-protest.html?smid=pl-share

Index

Milton Keynes UK
Ingram Content Group UK Ltd.
UKHW051854071024
449327UK00025B/1951

9 780367 583996